Casebook on Ethical Issues in International Health Research

Editors:

Richard Cash
Daniel Wikler
Abha Saxena
Alexander Capron

Associate editor:

Reva Gutnick

Editorial guidance provided by
Astrid Stuckelberger and Philippe Chastonay, University of Geneva

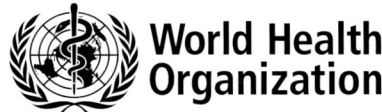

WHO Library Cataloguing-in-Publication Data

Casebook on ethical issues in international health research / edited by Richard Cash ... [et al].

1.Ethics, Research. 2.Research - standards. 3.Health services research. 4.Research design. 5.Case reports. I.Cash, Richard. II.Wikler, Daniel. III.Saxena, Abha. IV.Capron, Alexander M. V.World Health Organization.

ISBN 978 92 4 154772 7   (NLM classification: W 20.5)

© World Health Organization 2009

All rights reserved. Publications of the World Health Organization can be obtained from WHO Press, World Health Organization, 20 Avenue Appia, 1211 Geneva 27, Switzerland (tel.: +41 22 791 3264; fax: +41 22 791 4857; e-mail: bookorders@who.int). Requests for permission to reproduce or translate WHO publications – whether for sale or for noncommercial distribution – should be addressed to WHO Press, at the above address (fax: +41 22 791 4806; e-mail: permissions@who.int).

The designations employed and the presentation of the material in this publication do not imply the expression of any opinion whatsoever on the part of the World Health Organization concerning the legal status of any country, territory, city or area or of its authorities, or concerning the delimitation of its frontiers or boundaries. Dotted lines on maps represent approximate border lines for which there may not yet be full agreement.

The mention of specific companies or of certain manufacturers' products does not imply that they are endorsed or recommended by the World Health Organization in preference to others of a similar nature that are not mentioned. Errors and omissions excepted, the names of proprietary products are distinguished by initial capital letters.

All reasonable precautions have been taken by the World Health Organization to verify the information contained in this publication. However, the published material is being distributed without warranty of any kind, either expressed or implied. The responsibility for the interpretation and use of the material lies with the reader. In no event shall the World Health Organization be liable for damages arising from its use.

The named authors alone are responsible for the views expressed in this publication.

Using this casebook

This casebook has been developed as a teaching tool for instructors and workshop leaders rather than as a textbook for students or workshop participants. There is no need for participants to have copies of the casebook: facilitators can provide participants with individual case studies and chapter introductions relevant to the research ethics topic being addressed. Individual case studies and chapter introductions relevant to the research ethics topic being addressed can be photocopied from the print version or downloaded from the WHO web site without additional permission from WHO, unless the planned use is in conjunction with commercial purposes. Please ensure that the WHO source is appropriately acknowledged. If you plan to publish, adapt or translate the materials, please contact WHO directly at the following email: pubrights@who.int

Printed in Hong Kong

Table of contents

Acknowledgements 8

Foreword 9

The editors 10

Introduction 11

Teaching Guide 15

The Case Studies 35

Chapter I

Defining "Research" 37

Introduction: When must an ethics committee's approval be sought?

    Case 1. SARS and airplane passengers 42

    Case 2. Evaluating sexual health and family planning programmes 43

    Case 3. A treatment for central nervous system conditions 44

    Case 4. Documenting the health conditions of an indigenous community 45

Chapter II

Issues in Study Design 47

Introduction: Designing scientifically (and ethically) sound studies

    Case 5. Referral of severely ill children to hospital 55

    Case 6. Negotiating safe sex practices 56

    Case 7. Investigating treatment recommendations 57

    Case 8. Testing a new HBV vaccine 58

    Case 9. Tuberculosis prevention in HIV-positive people 59

    Case 10. Developing a vaccine for malaria 60

    Case 11. Should race be listed as a risk factor? 62

    Case 12. Short-course AZT to prevent mother-to-child transmission of HIV 63

    Case 13. Testing an ayurvedic medicine for malaria 65

    Case 14. Evaluating the use of traditional medicines for diarrhoea 67

    Case 15. Twin registry genetics 68

Case 16. Observing newborn care practices 69

Case 17. Compassionate intervention during an observational study.. 70

See also:

    Case 3. A treatment for central nervous system conditions

    Case 21. Pregnancy in health research

    Case 27. Micronutrient supplementation for pregnant women

    Case 42. Determining who constitutes the community

    Case 43. Evaluation research on a disability rehabilitation programme

Chapter III

Harm and Benefit..71

Introduction: Are research benefits and harms fairly distributed?

    Case 18. Rotavirus vaccine 76

    Case 19. Pneumonia vaccine trial... 78

    Case 20. Early termination of a trial 79

    Case 21. Pregnancy in health research... 80

    Case 22. Acting in the face of conflicting evidence 81

See also:

    Case 7. Investigating treatment recommendations

    Case 10. Developing a vaccine for malaria

    Case 11. Should race be listed as a risk factor?

    Case 13. Testing an ayurvedic medicine for malaria

    Case 28. Breastfeeding and mother-to-child HIV transmission

    Case 38. Mental health problems of survivors of mass violence

Chapter IV

Voluntary Informed Consent..83

Introduction: Is consent to research voluntary, knowing, and competent?

    Case 23. Testing high doses of vitamin A on children.. 92

    Case 24. Breast cancer in South Asia... 93

    Case 25. Testing a microbicide 95

    Case 26. A study to determine the value of postoperative radiotherapy 97

    Case 27. Micronutrient supplementation for pregnant women 98

Case 28. Breastfeeding and mother-to-child HIV transmission 100

Case 29. Humanized mice 102

Case 30. Donations for stem-cell research 103

Case 31. Researching health care practices and needs in an elderly population 104

See also:

    Case 1. SARS and airplane passengers

    Case 2. Evaluating sexual health and family planning programs

    Case 6. Negotiating safe sex practices

    Case 7. Investigating treatment recommendations

    Case 37. Testing a malaria vaccine

    Case 57. Testing a treatment for schizophrenia

Chapter V
Standard of Care 105

Introduction: Whose standard?

Case 32. Testing a new HIV vaccine 110

Case 33. Short-course antiretroviral therapy in pregnant women 112

Case 34. Use of quinacrine for non-surgical sterilization 113

Case 35. Investigation of vaginal microbicides 115

See also:

    Case 8. Testing a new HBV vaccine

    Case 9. Tuberculosis prevention in HIV-positive people

    Case 12. Short-course AZT to prevent mother-to-child HIV transmission

    Case 24. Breast cancer in South Asia

Chapter VI
Obligations to Participants and Communities 117

Introduction: How far do researchers' and sponsors' duties extend?

Case 36. Observational study of cervical cancer 124

Case 37. Testing a malaria vaccine 126

Case 38. Mental health problems of survivors of mass violence 128

Case 39. A longitudinal study of rotavirus incidence among young children 130

Case 40. Testing a vaccine for childhood cholera 132

Case 41. Impact of civil war on health systems 133

Case 42. Determining who constitutes the community 134

Case 43. Evaluation research on a disability rehabilitation programme 136

Case 44. Clinical benefits of an immune-modifying supplement in HIV therapy 138

Case 45. Genetic research on an island population 139

See also:

    Case 5. Referral of severely ill children to hospital

    Case 6. Negotiating safe sex practices

    Case 7. Investigating treatment recommendations

    Case 8. Testing a new HBV vaccine

    Case 10. Developing a vaccine for malaria

    Case 13. Testing an ayurvedic medicine for malaria

    Case 21. Pregnancy in health research

    Case 24. Breast cancer in South Asia

    Case 54. Health promotion survey research on a commercial farm

Chapter VII
Privacy and Confidentiality 141

Introduction: Who controls access to information?

Case 46. Studying Nevirapine in West Africa 146

Case 47. The quality of care in a family welfare programme 147

Case 48. Responding when study findings are challenged 148

Case 49. Determining post-abortion complication levels 149

Case 50. Evaluating the cost-benefit ratio of long-term care services 151

Case 51. Research on an identifiable population 152

Case 52. Case-control study of vasectomy and prostate cancer 153

Case 53. Studying health-seeking behaviour 154

Case 54. Health promotion survey research on a commercial farm 155

Case 55. Interviewing child domestic helpers in sub-Saharan Africa 157

See also:

    Case 1. SARS and airplane passengers

    Case 25. Testing a microbicide

    Case 45. Genetic research on an island population

Chapter VIII
Professional Ethics 159
Introduction: What to do when loyalties are divided?
How should research misbehaviour be defined and policed?

- Case 56. Testing delivery methods for a hormonal contraceptive 165
- Case 57. Testing a treatment for schizophrenia 166
- Case 58. Budget reviews by research ethics committees 167
- Case 59. Determining the workforce costs of the AIDS epidemic 168
- Case 60. Action research on involuntary resettlement.. 170
- Case 61. Victimizing the system or a victim of it?.. 172
- Case 62. Truth and consequences 174
- Case 63. The curious career of Dr Taylor.. 175
- Case 64. Whose idea is it, anyway?... 177

See also:

    Case 3. A treatment for central nervous system conditions

Glossary 179
Suggested readings and resources 193
Appendix 208

Acknowledgements

This casebook is the result of a collaborative effort titled "the Research Ethics Training Project" between the World Health Organization and the University of Geneva undertaken with the generous financial support of Réseau universitaire international de Genève/Geneva International Academic Network (RUIG/GIAN).

Many people have shared their time, energy and expertise in the development of this casebook. Philippe Chastonay and Astrid Stuckelberger of the Department of Social and Community Health at the Faculty of Medicine of the University of Geneva were involved in the initial brainstorming session that led to the generation of resources for the development and publication of the casebook. Although the idea for a casebook had originally been discussed in 2004, Dr Chastonay and Dr Stuckelberger's support was very instrumental in securing resources to allow the project to move forward from idea to reality. We are indebted to them for their initial and ongoing enthusiasm for the project. We would also like to acknowledge Daniel Warner of the Graduate Institute of International Studies in Geneva, who has been an important partner and collaborator in the project.

We acknowledge with gratitude those who have suggested or contributed case studies: James Hodge, Lawrence Gostin, Dirce Guilhem, Brooke Ronald Johnson, Neha Madhiwalla, Julie Milstein, Katherine Shapiro, Astrid Stuckelberger and Fabio Zicker. Case studies developed and contributed by Nancy Kass, Joan Atkinson, Liza Dawson and Andrea Ruff of the Johns Hopkins University Bloomberg School of Public Health and Johns Hopkins Berman Institute of Bioethics raise many important ethical issues and we are pleased to acknowledge their contributions to this casebook. The National Human Genome Research Institute has kindly provided permission for one of their case studies to be adapted and included here. We would also like to acknowledge the case studies developed by workshop participants in the UNDP-UNFPA-WHO-World Bank Special Programme of Research, Development and Research Training in Human Reproduction (HPR) in Bangkok, Thailand, 2004.

Participants in research ethics courses and workshops have used and commented on the case studies, and their input has allowed us to improve them greatly. Marie-Charlotte Bouësseau, Andreas Reis, Enrique Ezcurra, Florencia Luna, and Susan Bull have facilitated case study based workshop discussions in Africa, Asia, Europe and North America, and have provided valuable feedback. In addition, the case studies were used as an online teaching tool in two web-based training modules developed as part of the RUIG/GIAN project. The participants in those discussions have shown us the value and potential for using case-based teaching online. The online discussions were possible because of the time and commitment of Joseph Ali, Susan Bull, Adnan Hyder, Amar Jesani, Nancy Kass, Paul Ndebele, Sarah Pouzevara, Mala Ramathan and Neema Sofaer. Finally, reviewers from around the world have taken time from their busy schedules to review the draft and provide helpful advice: Clement Adebamowo, Zulfiqar Bhutta, Leonardo de Castro, Ames Dhai, Emmanuel Kabengele, Bebe Loff, Nicole Mamotte, Jens Mielke, Christina Torres, Sheryl Vanderpoel and Douglas Wassenaar. Maria Hirtle, Dominique Sprumont and others engaged in the TREE for Africa Project provided valuable feedback on both the teaching guide and the case studies.

In the early phases of the project, editorial and organizational support was provided by Emily Kaditz of Harvard University. Sona Ajit Chikarmane, Milena Petranovic and Giulia Reichmann contributed their writing and organizational skills while doing internships with the Ethics Review Committee Secretariat of WHO. We would like to thank Stefan Gutnick Allen for the cover concept and original cover design, Tushita Bosonet, Chris Burgisser and Aline Pavia of Tushita Graphic Vision for the final design of the entire casebook, and Christopher Black of WHO for assisting with the photographs used in the publication. Thank you also to technical editor Tara Satyanand. As project staff, Reva Gutnick has served as an invaluable associate editor.

It has been our pleasure and our honour to work with so many capable and dedicated people and we extend our thanks to each.

March 2009

Boston, Massachusetts	Richard Cash
	Dan Wikler
Geneva, Switzerland	Abha Saxena
Los Angeles, California	Alex Capron

Foreword

For the World Health Organization, research is a vital ingredient for improved global health. Our dedication to producing and using knowledge to improve human health is itself grounded on an ethical commitment: that such research is carried out ethically and offers the prospect of raising the standard of health for everyone.

One of the essential components of health research is a strong set of ethical standards, well understood and applied by research teams and sponsors. Examination of, and education about, the ethical issues raised by health research has been an important part of WHO's work for many years. As we step up our involvement with health research, it is thus important that we also increase our efforts within the Organization and with our collaborating centres and other groups at country and regional levels to ensure that ethical standards are met in all fields of health research – from initial trials of new technologies to epidemiologic studies to research on health systems.

These efforts are especially important in resource poor settings, where the need for locally applicable research findings is a foremost concern. As sponsors increase their funding of such research, it is crucial that local researchers who initiate or collaborate on such studies be able to identify and respond appropriately to the ethical issues they raise. Likewise, research ethics committees must be prepared to provide appropriate oversight to make sure that research projects are well designed and executed. Helping those who fund, carry out and review health research to deal with the ethical aspects is a matter of particular importance to WHO's departments of Research Policy and Cooperation and Ethics, Equity, Trade and Human Rights and to our in-house Ethics Review Committee, which has taken the lead in the development of the present casebook.

This book aims to help investigators, ethics review committee members, health authorities, and others to play their respective roles in the ethical conduct of research. Rather than take a didactic approach, the book is set up to provide cases – based on actual research studies – which can be read by individuals or discussed in group settings. Thinking one's way through the problems raised by such case studies has been shown both to be an extremely effective means of learning to understand and apply general ethical principles and to provide good preparation for dealing with the real world of health research.

Timothy Evans, D.Phil., M.D.
Assistant Director General
Information, Evidence and Research

The editors

Richard A. Cash MD, MPH, is a Senior Lecturer in the Department of Global Health and Population at the Harvard School of Public Health (HSPH). He is the Director of the Program on Ethical Issues in Global Health Research at HSPH. Dr Cash has been involved in international health for over 40 years as a researcher, a funder and developer of health research projects, and as a visiting faculty at a number of schools of public health around the world. He has conducted numerous research ethics workshops throughout Latin America, Africa, and Asia. Dr Cash began his research career in what is now Bangladesh where he and his colleagues conducted the first clinical trials of Oral Rehydration Therapy (ORT) for the treatment of diarrhoea. In 2006 he was awarded the prestigious Prince Mahidol Award in Thailand for his work on ORT.

Daniel Wikler, PhD, is Mary B. Saltonstall Professor of Population Ethics in the Department of Global Health and Population at the Harvard School of Public Health. Together with colleagues across the campus, he created the Harvard Program in Ethics and Health, addressing ethical issues involving health arising at the population and global levels. His research addresses ethical issues in global health, including health resource allocation, health measurement, and public health policy. Among numerous other publications, he is author, along with three fellow philosophers, of *From Chance to Choice: Genes and Justice*, published by Cambridge University Press. Prof. Wikler was co-founder and second president of the International Association of Bioethics. He served as the first "staff ethicist" at the World Health Organization in Geneva.

Abha Saxena MD has been managing the Research Ethics Review Committee of the World Health Organization in Geneva, Switzerland since 2002. Trained as an anaesthesiologist, she was a faculty member and Professor at the All India Institute of Medical Sciences, New Delhi, India, before joining WHO in 2001. As a medical practitioner, she was actively engaged for 20 years in hospital and community-based research. At WHO, in addition to running a dynamic research ethics committee, she conducts short training programmes in research ethics not only for WHO staff, but also in several African and Asian countries, using many of the case studies that are included in this casebook.

Alex Capron holds the Scott H. Bice Chair in Healthcare Law, Policy and Ethics in the Gould School of Law at the University of Southern California where he is also Professor of Law and Medicine at the Keck School of Medicine, and Co-Director of the Pacific Center for Health Policy and Ethics. Prof. Capron served as the first Director of Ethics, Trade, Human Rights and Health Law at the World Health Organization in Geneva. He was the Executive Director of the President's Commission for the Study of Ethical Problems in Medicine and Biomedical and Behavioral Research, and subsequently served as Chair of the Biomedical Ethics Advisory Committee of the U.S. Congress and as a member of the National Bioethics Advisory Commission. Prof. Capron has been President of the International Association of Bioethics, President of the American Society of Law, Medicine and Ethics, and Vice President of the Council for International Organizations of Medical Sciences (CIOMS). He has published widely on ethical, legal and social issues in biomedical research, health care and public health.

Introduction

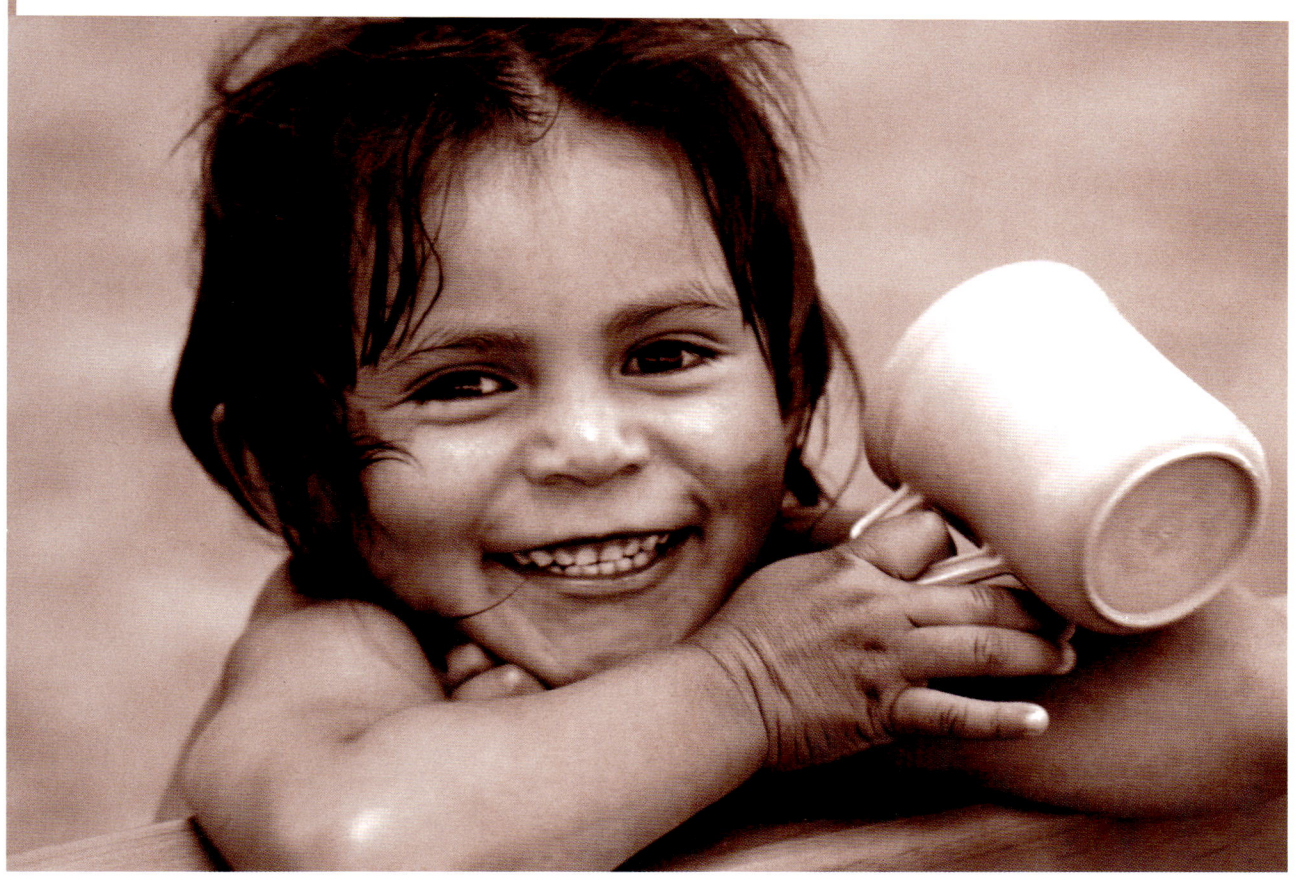

© WHO/ Photolibrary

Introduction

This casebook collects 64 case studies, each of which raises an important and difficult ethical issue connected with planning, reviewing, or conducting health-related research. The book's purpose is to contribute to thoughtful analysis of these issues by researchers and members of research ethics committees (RECs, known in some places as ethical review committees or institutional review boards), particularly those involved with studies that are conducted or sponsored internationally.

This collection is envisioned principally as a tool to aid educational programmes, from short workshops on research ethics to in-service learning for scientists and REC members, to formal degree or certificate courses. In such settings, instructors will typically select a number of case studies that will be distributed to the participants to provoke and focus discussion. (To assist those using these case studies in their classrooms and workshops, a teaching guide has been included.) Individuals who want to stimulate their own thinking about research ethics or to become more familiar with a range of real-world dilemmas in international health research, especially in developing countries, may also benefit from perusing this book, either on topics of special interest to them or as a whole.

The Case Studies

The case studies have been kept short (generally no more than two pages) and include only those descriptive background details that are relevant to the issue under discussion. While careful analysis will often reveal that more than one issue is raised by a case, each study is centred on one or two ethical problems. Cases are grouped in chapters based on the principal ethical questions that they address, but the table of contents suggests secondary categories under which the cases may also be fruitfully studied. In turn, as readers or course organizers become familiar with particular cases, they might want to re-assign them under further headings to take account of the additional issues that seem important to them. The arrangement of the cases (including the list of principal issues as delineated by the topical chapter headings) is intended to facilitate, not restrict, creative use of these materials.

The cases in this collection were not invented. Rather, each was drawn from one or more actual research projects. Some might seem familiar because they were controversial enough to prompt ethical debate in the news media or scientific journals, while others concern issues that have received less attention – but are not therefore less important. The names in the case studies and other topical information (such as dates and locations) have been changed so readers can focus on the ethical dilemmas. Some cases that were set in specific geographical contexts have been moved elsewhere by changing details to make them more useful in a particular educational setting. The descriptions are usually generic enough that readers can imagine what they would do if the research were proposed in their own locale. In some other cases, however, a specific disease being discussed is only found in a particular country or region, so that fact can't be changed, though such cases have also been edited to remove superfluous identifying details.

The Background

The publication of these materials by the World Health Organization (WHO) reflects its long-standing leadership in public health and biomedical research, especially on vaccines and drugs for the so-called "neglected diseases". In these activities, WHO works in partnership with its 193 Member States, other intergovernmental bodies, and nongovernmental organizations such as groups that deliver health care, foundations that sponsor research, research centres, and pharmaceutical companies. The growing complexity of such research – which can involve public-private partnerships, coordination of collaborators from diverse institutions and multiple countries, sponsors located far from the communities that host the research, growing commercial sponsorship of research, and the collection (and possible removal to distant repositories) of biological samples – has been accompanied by increased international attention to ethical problems. At the heart of this increased concern is the recognition that health-related studies have the potential to benefit the communities and populations involved – but can also harm them. The possibility of harm is especially great in settings where research participants are socially and economically vulnerable, poor and illiterate, and where they lack other access to health care.

All research projects supported by WHO are scrutinized by the WHO Research Ethics Review Committee (ERC) or by one of the WHO regional or country-level research ethics committees. In addition to its activities in developing guidance on research ethics and in reviewing research protocols, the ERC Secretariat organizes educational programmes for WHO staff at headquarters, and for WHO regional and country offices who are responsible for developing and overseeing research, and for members of the ERC itself. In reviewing research projects, the ERC Secretariat has also become aware of settings (especially but not exclusively in low-resource countries) where more education on research ethics would be helpful for researchers and the committees that provide ethical and scientific review of projects.

In its own educational programmes on research ethics, the ERC Secretariat has made extensive use of case studies, with case-based discussions guided by WHO's own staff and by external experts, especially colleagues from the Harvard School of Public Health (HSPH). The HSPH Program on Ethical Issues in International Health Research began holding an annual one-week workshop on research ethics in 1999. From the beginning, participants have been equally divided between developed and developing country scientists, researchers, administrators, and members of RECs and have been from governments, universities, and nongovernmental organizations. The workshops introduce participants to important (and sometimes controversial) concepts in research ethics through a mix of lectures and case study discussions. Although both methods are necessary, the HSPH organizers found that the case studies, which encourage participants to draw on – and then examine and defend – their own understanding of ethically acceptable actions, provided a safeguard against the imposition of cultural biases that may colour lecture-based sessions. Although people are sometimes reticent to question a lecturer, they are more likely to be willing to share their views about practical situations with which they are familiar. Moreover, analyzing case studies helps participants to move beyond generalities and to formulate concrete responses to dilemmas, just as researchers and REC members must do in practice. This collection of teaching cases has emerged from the HSPH and WHO workshops held around the world over nearly a decade, supplemented with ideas and cases suggested by many colleagues.

Teaching Guide

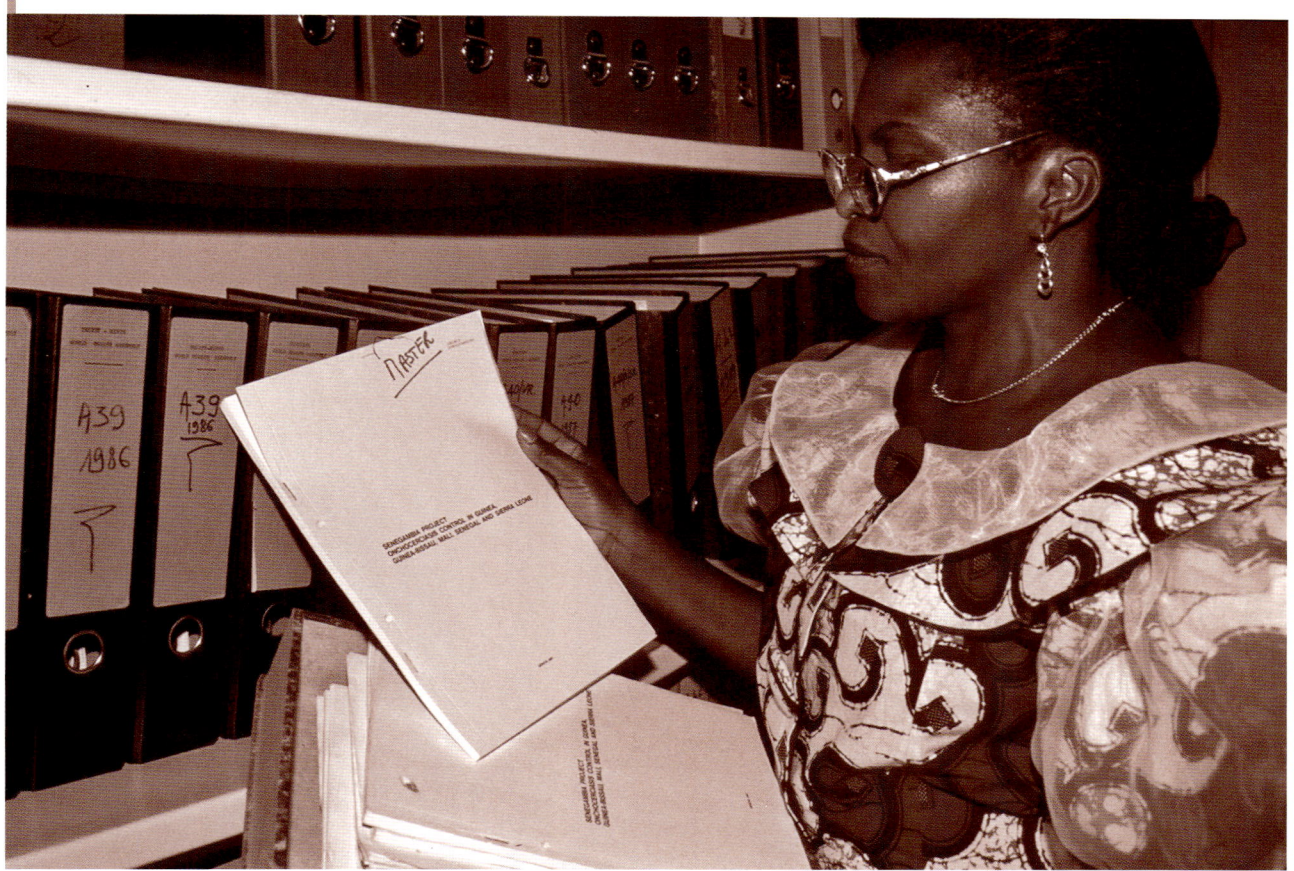

© WHO/TDR/Crump

Teaching Guide

Introduction

This brief teaching guide is intended as an aide to those using these case studies in their teaching or training workshops.

The guide first addresses the **process** of teaching case studies. Case-based teaching differs significantly from traditional lectures and, therefore, requires a different approach and additional skills. Because case-based teaching is typically used to enrich a learning experience by actively engaging students or workshop participants in structured discussions, one of the most important skills needed is the ability to lead a case study discussion. This guide offers some suggestions on how to do this well.

Second, the teaching guide addresses the **content** of the case studies by identifying some of the main issues in the case studies that the facilitator[1] should be aware of. The guide also suggests some questions that the facilitator can raise in order to encourage a thoughtful discussion of the issues. In some situations, the facilitator may have experience in using case studies to teach research ethics and can readily draw upon examples and counter-examples, guidelines and regulations to stimulate debate and discussion. More typically perhaps, the facilitator will have some background in research ethics and would like a little guidance on how to incorporate case studies in teaching the subject.

This guide also includes a list of additional resources for case-based teaching focused on articles dealing specifically with how to use case studies. In addition, the casebook itself includes a suggested reading list with links to international research ethics guidelines and numerous review articles. Finally, a glossary of medical, health and research terms is provided.

Using this casebook

This casebook has been developed as a teaching tool for instructors and workshop leaders rather than as a textbook for students or workshop participants. There is no need for participants to have copies of the casebook: facilitators can provide participants with individual case studies and chapter introductions relevant to the research ethics topic being addressed. Individual case studies and chapter introductions relevant to the research ethics topic being addressed can be photocopied from the print version or downloaded from the WHO web site without additional permission from WHO, unless the planned use is in conjunction with commercial purposes. Please ensure that the WHO source is appropriately acknowledged. If you plan to publish, adapt or translate the materials, please contact WHO directly at the following email: pubrights@who.int

---

[1] The term 'facilitator' is used here – instead of the term 'professor', 'teacher', 'instructor' or 'leader' – to emphasize that the faculty's role in case-based classes and workshops centres on enabling participants to utilize the case studies in an educationally enriching fashion. By using the term 'facilitator' we do not mean to introduce an additional person besides the professor or other leader of the course or training session, but merely to stress the difference in teaching method from a typical class.

Teaching Guide

Leading case-based discussions: the process

The role of the facilitator: helping participants learn through active engagement

In a typical lecture-based learning environment the focus is on the lecturer and the material he or she presents. Case-based teaching shifts the focus to the participants. The goal is for participants to *learn through actively engaging with the case studies*. Participants are encouraged to apply knowledge, reasoning, and their experiences and contexts to a real-life situation (the case study) and to learn from each others' responses. The role of the instructor or lecturer changes from being the expert who provides answers to that of a facilitator who encourages structured discussion among participants. In this section, we offer some suggestions for doing this.

At the outset, it is important to acknowledge that some teachers may feel that in facilitating a discussion, rather than delivering a lecture, they are not fulfilling their professional responsibility. This may be particularly true when there is a personal, professional or cultural expectation that a teacher's role is to provide "the answers". Case-based teaching, while less reliant on an obvious display of facilitators' expertise, actually places greater demands on their skills and knowledge than does straightforward lecturing. First, a thorough understanding of the subject matter is required so that the facilitator will be able to spot important points raised in a discussion even when they emerge in an unfamiliar fashion or in terms that may differ from those used by other experts. Second, special skills are needed to provide a supportive environment for students to develop their own analyses of the cases in a manner that is thorough and well-focused. You will, in short, be using your expertise, but sharing it in a less direct way as you encourage participants to address a range of ideas and to add to these by bringing in their own ethical reasoning and perspectives.

Being comfortable with cases that permit debate and disagreement

The case studies included here do not have easy or ready answers. They were chosen precisely because situations in which reasonable people can disagree about the right course of action are better suited for stimulating thinking than those about which everyone would agree. But teaching with these "open-ended" cases requires practice and skill. For example, there is no single correct answer regarding the extent of researchers' or sponsors' responsibility to provide tuberculosis care to participants in an HIV vaccine trial when screening of potential trial participants reveals that some are suffering from TB. You may have reached your own conclusion on the level and type of treatment that is owed, but the answer to this question is neither obvious nor self-evident, and it is important not to take sides by dismissing alternatives. Leading the participants towards your own conclusion or taking sides risks shutting down the discussion as participants may seek to please you by searching for what they think you regard as the 'right' answer. Meanwhile, they will not benefit from the potential of case-based discussion to motivate careful thinking and problem-solving, including articulating justifications for their conclusions.

Being comfortable with cases that permit debate and disagreement will allow you to both recognize that the ethical issues in the cases often pose dilemmas without easy answers and to help participants to recognize this as well. In addition to the questions at the end of each case study, there are a number of others that encourage the type of analytical discussion that the case studies are designed to elicit. Again, using the example of tuberculosis treatment in an HIV vaccine trial:

- Which points in the international guidance documents such as the CIOMS *International Ethical Guidelines*[1] or the *Declaration of Helsinki*[2] address the question of researchers' responsibility to treat conditions other than those that are the object of the study?

---

[1] Council for International Organizations of Medical Sciences (CIOMS). International Ethical Guidelines for Biomedical Research Involving Human Subjects. Geneva, Switzerland: Council for International Organizations of Medical Sciences (CIOMS), 2002. http://www.cioms.ch (accessed 9 May 2008)

[2] World Medical Association. Declaration of Helsinki: Ethical Principles for Medical Research Involving Human Subjects. Helsinki, Finland: World Medical Association, 1964. Most recent revised and updated version 2008. http://www.wma.net/e/ethicsunit/helsinki.htm (accessed 5 June 2009)

- Are there different ways that the guidelines can be interpreted and, if so, which ethical principles will help to resolve the question of responsibility?

- Does the context where the trial is taking place matter? More specifically, would people in your own community expect or need more from research and the researchers than those in more developed countries?

- Do, or should, participants in clinical trials have a right to benefit from their participation by obtaining much-needed medical care?

Preparing to use a case study

A facilitator should aim to select case studies that allow participants to concretely apply their understanding to the topic of the course module or workshop. Such cases offer an excellent opportunity for sharing and debating perspectives of immediate relevance across

- cultures (e.g. various approaches to individual signed consent),

- disciplines (e.g. a lawyer's analytic approach may raise significantly different issues than an anthropologist's),

- interests (e.g. a sponsor may raise different concerns than a ministry of health policy-maker or a community representative).

> In choosing a case study, consideration should be given to the cultural context in which the case study will be used. Some case studies will be more difficult to teach in certain contexts than others and may even be inappropriate. Sensitivity to community norms (cultural, religious, gender) may rule out the use of particular cases either because the cases may seem irrelevant or because they may be considered too sensitive.

It is always a good idea to provide participants with a copy of the case study in advance of the session when it will be discussed and to ask them to read and think about it beforehand. In some circumstances, it may also be appropriate to give participants an additional assignment (such as preparing an informed consent form for the clinical trial discussed in a case study, or a memorandum listing the relevant issues and proposing how to resolve them) that can be used as a starting point for discussion when the case is presented.

Case studies can be discussed either before or after the participants have been introduced (through a lecture or a discussion) to the substantive issues being addressed in the workshop or class session.

- When a case study is used before a lecture or seminar discussion introducing the topic or issue, participants will draw on their existing knowledge to examine the case study and identify areas where they need more background both to fully understand the issues and to make informed suggestions on how to address them. Participants can then be provided with additional resources (theory, relevant current debates, existing guidelines which may be applicable, examples of various practices), or when circumstances permit, participants may be encouraged to seek out appropriate resources for themselves. To aid participants, the material covered in such additional resources may be reviewed in a lecture given by the facilitator or another expert who has been invited to address the class or workshop on the issues raised by the case study.

- When a case study is used after the participants have obtained some relevant background through advanced reading, a lecture, or a seminar discussion of the general issues that will be raised by the case, the participants would generally be expected to apply or relate the material to the case study.

Each approach has its advantages. Starting with a case study is likely to engage the participants more than starting with a lecture; it may also cause them to be more receptive to ethical concepts and guidelines which they will then recognize as potentially helpful in resolving the issues that arose in their discussion of the alternatives presented by the case study. On the other hand, starting with a lecture and/or a review of background materials is likely to improve the quality of the discussion and to give the students a more immediate sense of mastery.

Whatever the timing of the case study, an important part of the facilitator's preparation is devising a good starting point for the case discussion. If the group is large (i.e. 20 or more participants), the discussion will probably be enhanced by dividing into small groups of 6 to 8 people and allowing 20-30 minutes for small group discussion before assembling into the large group. (For example, in a workshop setting, the small group discussion could take place over breakfast.) The facilitator should remind the small groups that everyone should express themselves and be respectful of other participants' comments; the facilitator can also walk among the groups to keep an eye on their progress and add a question or comment if the group seems to need additional input. Some participants may be reluctant to express their ideas or to argue a point in a large group but feel more comfortable speaking in a more intimate setting; after exploring their ideas in the small group, they may feel emboldened to speak in a larger audience.

The introduction you provide to a case study – such as the first question you ask or the exercise you assign – will serve to guide the subsequent discussion. For example, if you would like workshop participants to explore the obligations owed to trial participants such as the type, level and duration of care before approaching issues of study design and informed consent, then your opening should be crafted to elicit responses about obligations. You may want to begin by initially asking questions specifically about obligations to those accepted into the trial before asking about obligations to those who contract the study disease, those who contract a different disease, or the ethics of treating a participant for the target disease but not her infant child. If there is immediate agreement on all the answers, gently probe a little further to determine where individual participants would draw the limits of these obligations; you can also explore the different ethical as well as human rights principles on which they are based. Only after a topic has reached an analytical depth you are satisfied with should you move onto the other issues in the case study. If participants raise other issues (such as study design or informed consent) in the course of the discussion on obligations, thank them and write these issues on a flip chart or whiteboard (so that the idea does not get lost) but indicate that these issues will be discussed later in the session.

One way to encourage discussion is to ensure that the initial question you raise is one that permits more than one single appropriate response. Continuing with the previous example, ask whether sponsors should provide treatment for tuberculosis in the HIV vaccine trial and if so, why? Rather than agreeing or disagreeing with any statements, follow up with a question such as: if 50% of trial participants are anticipated to be in need of the treatment, in addition to those who get treatment for HIV/AIDS, might sponsors find these obligations too onerous? Based on expense and a possibility of conflict, what if the sponsor would therefore likely decide to abandon the vaccine trial, or to take it to another setting where the added requirements wouldn't be imposed? And if this might happen, should there be no demand for such treatment? Try to anticipate what the responses might be; thinking about follow-up questions in advance will help you to guide the participants to a deeper analysis and awareness. Anticipating the flow of the discussion will also allow you to seek out pertinent examples, topical debates, and relevant articles in advance. These can be used to stimulate the discussion or take it in another direction when it is timely to do so.

Be prepared to stimulate discussion by *posing challenges to viewpoints and positions that you agree with* in addition to questioning those with which you disagree. You will encounter participants who share your views but whose reasons for holding these views do not offer logical support for them.

If you challenge them to re-think their arguments, they will gain knowledge and skills that can serve them well when faced with other ethical dilemmas in their future work.

Guidelines for facilitating a group discussion

While each facilitator will bring his or her own skills to the role, we offer a few brief suggestions here.

1. Provide affirming and encouraging comments as these will promote a safe and supportive environment that will help to overcome any initial reluctance of some participants to speak. Encourage everyone to be supportive rather than competitive with each other as this will promote a full and lively discussion.

2. Try to get many different people to speak when the case is discussed; move the discussion around from left to right and front to back so that all feel that they are active participants. When a speaker's voice is too soft, repeat the comment or question.

3. In order to discourage "in-groups" and "out-groups", treat all participants fairly and equally even if some are known to you. When speaking, address the entire group, not just the speaker or questioner as everyone is part of the audience.

4. The language used in the classroom or workshop may be the second or third language of some of the participants. Some participants may be struggling to communicate and may be abrupt in their communication as a result of language and not intent. When that occurs, you can reiterate the heart of the participant's comment; such rephrasing will not only allow others to comprehend the point and provide them with a model of how to make a point but will also allow you to confirm that the original speaker's idea has been correctly understood.

5. Discourage participants from bringing in private debates; rather, encourage them to open the discussion to everyone.

6. Avoid and deflect any personal attacks.

7. Assist participants in looking at the same issue from a number of different perspectives.

8. Feel free to modify the case study by adding more information or changing certain details when that will help the discussion move forward.

9. Encourage participants to move back and forth between the case studies and the research guidelines and other material they may have read or been presented in order to build the most comprehensive knowledge. Use phrases like, "What about if…", "That's a good point but how does it fit with…", "Here's an example of a drug trial where the opposite was done and …", "Can you think of a local example or an example from your own experience…?"

10. Encourage participants to speak succinctly and directly.

11. Discussions can take unexpected turns – both for the better and for the worse. Try to determine which is which, and be flexible enough to follow the good leads and astute enough to gently re-direct the discussion if the diversion is not useful.

12. As the discussion progresses, from time to time summarize what has been covered in order to assure participants that learning is indeed happening. Case studies, which can be full of dilemmas and don't have ready answers, can leave participants feeling frustrated that nothing has been resolved even though there has been much talk. A summary in which attention is drawn to the key insights can reassure participants, move discussion forward to the next points to be addressed, and provide a useful wrap-up for the session. A group discussion of a case can, at its best, impart insights as effectively as an expert "Socratic" lecture, i.e. one in which the lecturer draws the insights out of the participants rather than offering them as part of a prepared talk.

Teaching Guide

Exploring the content of each chapter

> This section is intended for discussion facilitators or leaders while the chapter introductions in the casebook itself are suitable for copying and sharing with students and workshop participants.

The case studies are organized into chapters based on the principal ethical issue raised in each study. Most raise additional dilemmas and can easily be used to raise more than one issue; the table of contents suggests ways for reassigning some cases among the existing categories. Facilitators may choose to identify cases that deal with a particular topic of interest, such as studies involving reproductive health or a phase II clinical trial or studies conducted in a particular geographical location.

While the chapter introductions provide important background material for participants in the workshop or class, the material provided here in this teaching guide is intended to help facilitators identify some of the main ethical issues chapter by chapter. The questions provided are intended to suggest how the ethical issues in the case studies can be approached in a discussion and some areas that the facilitator may wish to prepare for in advance of the discussion. Although there are many more questions, readings and examples than are provided here, we hope that these prove to be a useful starting point.

Chapter I: What is research?

This chapter encourages workshop or classroom participants to consider two distinctions: first, research with human participants as distinct from medical treatment and, second, the differences between research and other activities involving some sort of investigation with human beings (e.g. evaluation, surveillance or audit). What is it that distinguishes each of these activities and leads only some (i.e. health research) to require approval by a research ethics committee? For example, does the level of risk to participants play a role in the decision to require ethical oversight? An exploration of these questions can lead quite naturally into a discussion of the mandate and authority of research ethics committees. The points below expand on these questions and can be used to encourage participants to consider the following:

- Why lines might need to be drawn between research, on the one hand, and medical treatment or public health activities, on the other.

  - Are such lines primarily useful for analytic purposes, or as a means of determining which activities need which types of ethical standards and oversight?

  - Is research inherently more risky than medical treatment or public health activities, and hence in need of oversight by people other than researchers, or can non-research activities pose equal or greater risks, and if so, are oversight mechanisms used for research relevant or irrelevant to reducing the risks of non-research activities?

- The differences in objectives, and hence of obligations, between medical treatment (the therapeutic or humanitarian mission) and health research (the knowledge generation mission). Awareness of such differences (or 'conflict of missions') is relevant for a number of reasons, prime among them is whether the trust of patients in the medical profession is endangered when a physician recruits a patient into a research study.

  - How should a physician engaged in health research ensure that a patient who is a 'potential research participant' is aware that a medical intervention is being undertaken to generate knowledge and not necessarily (or, at least, not solely) to advance the patient's individual health interests? What does a patient need to know before becoming a participant and how and by whom should this information be relayed?

- What is the role of informed consent? That is, what purpose is it supposed to serve? Why would (most) research be unethical without informed consent?

- Are there circumstances when it would be inappropriate – even wrong – to enrol patients as research participants? Is this true even when the patients would be willing to participate, if asked?

- If potential participants are vulnerable – perhaps because they have limited or no access to appropriate health care, as is often the case in developing countries – are there additional considerations that need to be taken into account? Does it make sense to describe patients from ethnic minorities or women and children as 'vulnerable', a term that is often used for people who are poor (or, more generally, residents of developing countries)?

- Some patients join research studies because they have no other way to get the care they need. Is their participation "voluntary"? Even if they understand the terms of the invitation to participate, should their consent be regarded as valid? Should the recruitment of these patients be carried out any differently? Do the various guidelines have anything to say on this? How would the ethical principle of 'respect for persons' be applied in this case?

- What role-confusion may researchers experience when working with patient-participants?

  - If a medical practitioner begins with the role of treating patients using the best known methods, then how is research, which uses unproven and possibly risky new interventions, justifiable?

  - Is it an ethical problem, or even a conflict of interest, for a physician to be paid for recruiting patients into a research study?

  - Does the determination of which body or committee should be charged with providing ethical review and oversight depend upon the objective of a particular activity? What considerations does a research ethics committee need to take into account in its review as opposed to considerations which ought to concern bodies that oversee medical practice?

- Compare research activities (including epidemiological research, operations research, formative research) with activities that also aim to produce information, such as public health surveillance, audit, and programme evaluation.

  - The common definition of research, which focuses on the production of 'generalizable knowledge', is intended to exclude the practice of medicine even though therapeutic and diagnostic interventions sometimes produce new information (especially about a particular patient) or amount to 'innovative treatment'. Does the same distinction hold between research and the practice of public health when activities such as public health surveys and disease surveillance may involve large numbers of observations and produce scientifically valid findings?

  - Advance review and approval were instituted for clinical trials and other biomedical studies because of the numerous instances where physicians and other scientists had overstepped ethical lines in carrying out research. Are the same requirements appropriate for public health research that is carried out by publicly accountable officials? What sorts of authorization, in terms of statutes or regulations, should be regarded as substitutes for the prior ethical review and individual informed consent mandated for clinical trials and comparable types of health research?

This chapter on defining research can also:

- Provide a starting point for examining research guidance documents such as the World Medical Association's *Declaration of Helsinki* (DoH),[1] the CIOMS *International Ethical Guidelines for Biomedical Research Involving Human Subjects*,[2] and the CIOMS *International Ethical Guidelines for Epidemiological Studies*,[3] since all address the tension between health research with human beings and medical treatment. The DoH was developed by the World Medical Association to address the ethical responsibilities of physicians when conducting research; both of the CIOMS international ethical guidelines documents are intended to elaborate the *Declaration* especially for use in developing country settings.

- Be used to explore the evolution of research ethics guidelines and the importance of separating research from medical practice; the preamble in each of the CIOMS guidance documents provides a good introduction for understanding what constitutes research.

- Provide concrete examples for exploring the mandate of a research ethics committee (REC) and therefore a good place to begin an initial training workshop for REC members. Facilitators may wish to provide additional examples of situations where it was either not clear whether the information being gathered was research or, for example, public health surveillance, and examples where research must be stopped and medical treatment provided.

Chapter II: Issues in Study Design

The proper design of research studies presents numerous scientific and management questions, such as the appropriateness of a study design to answer the hypothesis, whether it has adequate statistical power to produce valid results, and the ability to achieve the sample size in a timely fashion. But the scientific design of a study can also raise significant ethical issues. For example, research in social psychology often relies on deception. In one famous series of experiments, research participants were placed in a group and were tested to see if their judgments were influenced by the opinions of other group members. However, unknown to the research participants, the group members were actually confederates of the research team whose statements were set by the experimental script.[4] According to the investigators, the study would have been impossible if they were required to disclose this deception in order to obtain informed consent. Instead, they argued, it would be ethical to wait to tell the research participants these facts as part of a 'debriefing' after they had participated in the experiment. A different kind of ethics-related design issue arises when research designs appear to be chosen specifically to ensure an outcome favourable to the study's sponsor. For example, to increase the chance that an investigative drug will prove superior to a rival treatment a clinical trial might use the latter at a subclinical dosage, or the endpoints chosen might be those known through preliminary trials to be particularly affected by the investigative drug rather than those of greater clinical importance.

International research carried out in developing or resource-poor countries requires that the research be sensitive to the social, cultural, political and economic context of the country and community in which the research will take place. The design of these studies should avoid exploiting the population; furthermore, there is growing consensus that research should contribute to expanding the capacities of the health systems in such countries and to reducing health disparities.

---

[1] WMA, op.cit., p.13.

[2] CIOMS, op.cit., p.13.

[3] Council for International Organizations of Medical Sciences (CIOMS). International Ethical Guidelines for Epidemiological Studies. Geneva, Switzerland: Council for International Organizations of Medical Sciences (CIOMS), 2009. http://www.cioms.ch (accessed 19 May 2009)

[4] Asch, S. E., Opinions and Social Pressure, *Scientific American*, 193: 31-35 (1955); Korn, J.H., Illusions of Reality: A History of Deception in Social Psychology, Albany, NY: State University of New York Press (1997), esp. pp. 76-80.

A recent monograph by Dr Patricia Marshall, *Ethical Challenges in Study Design and Informed Consent for Health Research in Resource-poor Settings*,[1] provides excellent background preparation for facilitating a discussion based on this chapter and is useful also for chapters 3 to 6. Her work draws attention to the centrality in designing ethical research, of paying attention to cultural contexts, health disparities, collaborative partnerships and capacity building, standards of care, and access to benefits derived from research. In addition, the case studies and commentaries in *Ethical Issues in International Biomedical Research: A Casebook*,[2] provide very useful background and real life examples that can be used to illustrate ideas raised in the classroom or workshop.

A number of issues are raised by the case studies in this chapter, including:

- The relationship between questionable science and ethics, and how an ethics committee should respond when asked to review a protocol that appears to be scientifically unsound, naïve, or inappropriate to the task. One viewpoint is that research ethics committees should be concerned primarily with ethical questions, referring questions of scientific soundness to others responsible for (and expert in) the particular field of scientific research. An alternative view is that 'bad science is bad ethics', even in studies that pose little or no risk to subjects, and that research ethics committees must therefore be concerned with scientific as well as ethical questions. A complicating factor is that in resource-poor settings it may be impractical to divide these responsibilities among multiple committees.

- Whether individual rights and protections are compromised by the research design when, for example, the risk-benefit ratio appears too high, when the research is conducted with an identifiable population or group which may be stigmatised or otherwise harmed by the results, or when the participants are not fully informed such as in a study design which uses deception or observation. The "Tearoom Trade" study, conducted by Laud Humphreys, is one of the most well-known studies in which an investigator disguised the purpose of the research from his subjects.[3] It may provide a useful example for a discussion concerning the trade-off between gaining scientific knowledge and respecting research participants. The article in the reading list by F. Van den Borne, entitled Using Mystery Clients to Assess Condom Negotiation in Malawi, is an excellent resource for understanding deception design and the rationale for 'mystery clients'.[4]

- Whether there are research designs which could yield quality results but are less risky for subjects or impose a smaller burden on them.

---

[1] Marshall PA. Ethical Challenges in Study Design and Informed Consent for Health Research in Resource-poor Settings. Geneva, Switzerland: WHO/TDR, 2007. https://www.who.int/tdr/publications/tdr-research-publications/ethical-challenges-study-design/pdf/ethical_challenges.pdf (accessed 30 August 2008)

[2] Lavery JV, Grady C, Wahl ER, Emanuel E (eds.). Ethical Issues in International Biomedical Research: a casebook. Oxford, UK: Oxford University Press, 2007.

[3] Humphreys L. Tearoom Trade: Impersonal Sex in Public Places. Chicago: Aldine Publishing Co., 1970.

[4] Van den Borne F. Using Mystery Clients to Assess Condom Negotiation in Malawi: Some Ethical Concerns. *Studies in Family Planning* 2007;38[4]. http://dx.doi.org/10.1111/j.1728-4465.2007.00144.x (accessed 25 August 2008)

- The question of justice when certain populations are excluded because of age, gender or an existing disease. These people may be spared the burden (if any) of the research, but the information obtained through the study may then not be as useful in treating people in these populations. Conversely, when participation in research would be likely to confer a net benefit for research participants, is it unfair to exclude members of these populations in order to strengthen the study design (e.g. when the inclusion of older patients, who are more likely to die of other causes, might obscure a modest but real extension of life among research participants who receive the experimental intervention)?

- What provision must be made for treatment and care of participants, their families and communities? Given that ethical guidelines generally operate at the level of broad principles, rather than specifying practical applications, how would one go about negotiating or determining the exact obligations regarding treatment for research subjects in light of the principles stated in the guidelines? Do the guidelines themselves provide adequate ethical justification for such obligations?

- Whether it is ethical to give the participants assigned to the control arm of a clinical trial a placebo, and if so, under what circumstances and contexts? Two important features of research design, equipoise and randomisation, can be explored through the case studies in this chapter. In addition to the articles in the suggested reading list for this chapter, and the basic ethics guidelines (such as the DoH and the CIOMS *International Ethical Guidelines*), both the previously cited *Ethical Issues in International Biomedical Research: A Casebook*,[1] and the *Ethical Challenges in Study Design and Informed Consent for Health Research in Resource-poor Settings*[2] monograph address the topic of using placebos in clinical trials.

- Whether traditional medicine can and should be tested and measured using western scientific research methodologies (as in Case Study 14, titled *Evaluating the Use of Traditional Medicines for Diarrhoea*). If not, then how can they be effectively researched? Is it ethical to test a traditional treatment when an effective allopathic alternative exists? Do the same standards apply – and if not, why not? Are the international guidelines in conflict with the testing and promotion of traditional and alternative treatments?

- Whether, to win approval from a research ethics committee, a study must be in line with the country's national priorities in health care and research. If the disease under study is not a high priority, or if citizens of that country will not be able to afford the treatment being tested, should the research be carried out there?

Chapter III: Harm and Benefit

Risk of harm to research participants is one of the most difficult issues that all stakeholders in the research process (researchers, sponsors, research institutions, host countries, research ethics committees and participants) must consider and weigh. What risks are acceptable to achieve the anticipated benefits? Who should be asked to accept these risks and why? Who should decide what level of risk is acceptable? In the context of research in developing countries, resolving the issues raised by such questions is crucial in ensuring ethical research.

---

[1] Lavery, op.cit., p. 21.

[2] Marshall, op.cit., p.20.

With research increasingly being conducted in developing countries, there has been a greater focus on the broad range of potential harms and benefits, and the special allocation issues that arise in contexts where many factors – poverty, a lack of access to healthcare, gender inequality and other vulnerabilities – need to be taken into consideration in weighing the harm-benefit ratio. How can one achieve the "optimal synergy between the development of new health technologies, on the one hand, and the promotion and protection of ethical and human rights principles, on the other ".[1] Recent clinical trials of microbicides for HIV prevention (such as those described in *Ethical Issues in International Biomedical Research: A Casebook*[2]) bring these issues to the forefront. The National Bioethics Advisory Commission report, *Ethical and Policy Issues in International Research: Clinical Trials in Developing Countries*,[3] can also be a useful resource for this chapter. Recent ethical guidance strongly suggests that the question of benefits is not only about benefits to individuals – although this remains important – but also benefits to families, communities and countries (for example, providing post-trial access to a successful intervention broadly rather than solely to the people who took part in the research). There is, as yet, little consensus on the extent of such obligations, and research ethics committees have to reach their own judgments.

When working with each of the case studies in this chapter, students or workshop participants will need to consider the following:

- The risk of participants being harmed either during the research process or once the results are disseminated. The risks to participants in social science research ought not be overlooked as, for example, the literature on research on violence against women aptly demonstrates.

- Whether any aspects of the research design generate unnecessary risks and, if so, what can be changed to provide subjects with greater protection?

- Whether the benefits to the participants, or to other future beneficiaries, warrant the risk of harm to this particular group of participants, their families and communities. What contextual factors or specificities need to be considered in each case study in order to make a decision as to whether the harm/benefit ratio is acceptable?

- If participants are informed of, understand, and accept the risks of a research study, does this release the research ethics committee of responsibility for approving what may be a risky trial? How should responsibility for adverse outcomes be apportioned among the scientists, the research subjects, and the research ethics committee? What do international guidelines and norms have to say on the just allocation of potential harms and benefits, particularly in research conducted in developing countries?

- Whether certain potential harms are ethically acceptable… What safeguards are in place – e.g. a data safety monitoring board (DSMB) – to monitor and stop trials should problematic results occur in each of the phases? What are the ethical responsibilities of a DSMB?

---

[1] Tarantola D, et al. Ethical considerations related to the provision of care and treatment in vaccine trials. Vaccine, 2007, 25:4863-4874.
http://dx.doi.org/10.1016/j.vaccine.2007.03.022 (accessed 25 August 2008)

[2] Lavery, op.cit. p. 21.

[3] National Bioethics Advisory Commission. Ethical and Policy Issues in International Research: Clinical Trials in Developing Countries, Volumes I and II. Bethesda, MD, USA: National Bioethics Advisory Commission, 2001.
http://bioethics.georgetown.edu/nbac/pubs.html (accessed 9 May 2008)

- What benefits are anticipated and do these outweigh the risks? What factors would you consider in determining the right balance? How are the risks and benefits allocated? Are there obligations which come with asking people to take risks and what are these? Are they to participants alone or to broader groups of people? In a country where participants may have little access to health care, are the obligations to provide benefits higher than they would be in a developed country?

- Can a potential trial benefit become an 'undue inducement' to participate? Is this a universal standard or contextual? If a potential participant who is aware that a trial entails high risk is given substantial amounts of money – or other goods or services – to "compensate" for the risk and then agrees to take part in the trial, is this unethical? Conversely, would it be unethical to seek out subjects willing to participate for a more modest reward? What ethical principles might one use to help reach a decision?

Chapter IV: Voluntary Informed Consent

The case studies in this chapter are intended not only to draw attention to the importance of informed consent, but to explore informed consent processes in the context of international health research. Numerous studies have shown that participants in research too often do not have an adequate understanding of the purpose of the research they are being asked to consent to, nor of its potential harms and benefits and the alternatives to participation. Because informed consent is mandatory in most research contexts, an important question becomes how to ensure that information about the research, and the participant's agreement to participate, is appropriately communicated. The case studies in this chapter encourage discussion of a range of alternatives.

- Contextual factors in countries and communities where international research is conducted make it highly inappropriate to try to export a standardized consent form from one country and context to another, especially from a developed to a developing country. But is it appropriate to export the requirement for individual informed consent itself? (As a facilitator teaching Case 24, you may wish to be familiar with the work of Love et.al., whose work is relevant to this case.[1])

- "Informed consent" is an ambiguous term: it could mean either that a potential subject has been informed about a clinical trial or that the subject has understood what he or she has been told, or both. In the context of treatment, the former seems to have been the original meaning, whereas in the context of research, the people introducing the term apparently had the latter meaning in mind. Should we therefore abandon the term and look instead for "consent based on adequate disclosure" and "comprehending consent," respectively? Should we call the process "understood consent" as a way of determining whether the participant can answer specific questions, either verbally or in writing, regarding the specifics of the study?

---

[1] Love RR., et al. Oophorectomy and Tamoxifen Adjuvant Therapy in Premenopausal Vietnamese and Chinese Women with Operable Breast Cancer. *Journal of Clinical Oncology*. 2002 May 15;20(10):2559-66.
http://jco.ascopubs.org/cgi/content/full/20/10/2559 (accessed 30 August 2008)

- Informed consent as an underlying principle of ethical research implies (and depends on) each research participant's ability to make a decision autonomously. However, culture, custom, or other factors having to do with safety or trust for example, may place a higher value on the prerogative of a community leader or a male head of household to make decisions for others. Individual autonomy may hold a much lower value and may even be seen as challenging an established structure. Students or workshop participants should be encouraged to think about the application of international guidelines and human rights principles – all of which require individual informed consent by competent persons – in local contexts. This may involve both looking at the concept of individual consent, as well as the process by which it can be negotiated in order to ensure that the research is possible.

- A signed informed consent form is generally seen as adequate assurance that the participant has understood and agreed to the research. However, rather than looking at informed consent as merely a signature that signals a person's agreement to participate, students or workshop participants can consider what it would mean, in theory and practice, to treat informed consent as a process that is sensitive to contextual specificities. Culturally appropriate ways of disclosing information about the research should be found, as should an appropriate way of manifesting true consent and assent. Marshall's *Ethical Challenges in Study Design and Informed Consent for Health Research in Resource-poor Settings*[1] draws attention to, and provides examples of, a wide range of issues relevant for informed consent, including comprehension of information, communication of risks, decisional authority to consent to research, community consultation, and awareness of, and sensitivity to, social position and power inequities.

- Informed consent challenges researchers to take the time necessary to learn about the community where they are planning to conduct research, for example:

  - how are concepts of health and disease explained in this community, and how are illnesses traditionally treated? Is there a concept of research, and if so, who is trusted to conduct research?

  - what role does the community leadership play in decision-making in areas such as this? Is it clear who the leaders are, and who represents the best interests of the community and of the individuals who are part of that community?

  - could perceived or actual dangers result from signing a consent form or having a signed copy in one's home? In some places, people have (naively or under duress) signed forms that led to the loss of their homes or land; to ask potential subjects in such a locale to sign an informed consent form may therefore be inappropriate. A different sort of example arises in research on violence against women; investigators must exercise a high degree of sensitivity, since anything that links subjects to such a study risks exposing them to further violence.

  - is the potential participant literate and able to read the information provided or is it important to provide the information in a more accessible manner?

  - who is, and who isn't, competent to sign on their own behalf and why? If people are found to be incompetent (on account, for example, of being a minor or having a mental handicap), do provisions exist to allow for their wishes to be taken into account?

[1] Marshall, op.cit., p.20.

Chapter V: Standard of Care

This chapter focuses on the heated debate in research ethics over whether a single, universal standard of care should be applied (i.e. participants in a clinical trial conducted in multiple locations would all receive the same care, even when care for non-participants differs greatly among the locations), or whether, taking socio-economic differences among locales into account, the standard of care changes as well. (Chapter VI on obligations to participants and communities raises additional related issues.)

The Nuffield Council on Bioethics report titled *The Ethics of Research Related to Healthcare in Developing Countries*[1] provides a good discussion of standards of care in developing country contexts and is suitable background for students and workshop participants. The report draws attention to the many ways that the research context adds complexities to what may initially seem like a fairly straightforward proposition – that equity requires that care for patients in health research should meet the 'highest possible standard' or care.

Some of the issues raised by the case studies in this chapter are as follows:

- What do international ethics documents say on the subject of placebos and what ethical reasoning do they provide? When an effective therapy exists, can the use of a placebo control ever be consistent with such documents' requirement that researchers and sponsors must provide the highest possible standard of care to all research participants?

- How is the "highest standard of care" defined? Compare these circumstances in which the treatment deemed best in wealthy countries:

  - is simply not feasible in a developing country context, e.g. because there are not adequate refrigeration or storage facilities, or because the drug supply chain does not operate well in a consistent fashion.

  - has not yet been approved for sale in the developing country, though it probably would be if it were submitted for approval.

  - is available in the developing country but only at high prices, or to a small elite, and though it could in practice be provided to all who need it, the cost (in money and/or in medical resources) would make this an unwise use of resources

  - has not be designated as the treatment of choice by the local ministry of health (whether for sound reasons or otherwise)

- If the prevailing standard of care is noticeably higher in a developed country (from where the investigator and/or sponsor come from) than in a developing country (where the research will be carried out),

  - is it ethical to provide the highest standard of care available anywhere in the world to the control arm *knowing* that others in the country with the same medical condition are not able to access that care? Might care at such a high level amount to an unfair inducement to participate in the research?

  - is it ethically preferable to provide – or not to provide – the highest standard of care to participants in the trial if there is no commitment (on the part of the research sponsor or the local health authorities) to continue to provide that level of care after the trial is finished?

---

[1] Nuffield Council on Bioethics. The Ethics of Research Related to Healthcare in Developing Countries. London, UK: Nuffield Foundation, 2002.
http://www.nuffieldbioethics.org/go/ourwork/developingcountries/introduction
(accessed 24 August 2008)

- would it ever be justified not to provide the highest standard of care to the control arm and instead to give them the local standard because that is what they would be getting if they weren't in the trial? Would doing so exploit an already vulnerable population and indicate that this population is of lesser value because its members live in a developing rather than a developed country where the highest standard is available to people like themselves?

- would it ever be justified not to provide the highest standard of care to the study participants when that standard would be so expensive or logistically difficult that requiring it would preclude testing a new therapy that would probably be very effective – albeit not as effective as the best therapy – when the new therapy would (if proven effective) be affordable for people in the test country, whereas the best therapy will not become available to the population for many years?

- is it ethical to test an intervention that is less than the highest standard against the highest standard, knowing that the intervention being tested is not likely to be as efficacious? How much less efficacious is acceptable? Would it be wrong to test such an intervention against the current best standard because the new intervention is likely to "fail" in such a trial, which would cause it to be rejected (even if it would "succeed" compared to a placebo and would offer the local population a better alternative than any now actually available to them)?

- if conducting such a trial would not be acceptable in a developed country, under what circumstances, if any, should it be approved by a research ethics committee in a developing country? What ethical principles or other factors should be considered?

Chapter VI: Obligations to Participants and to the Community

There is little consensus on exactly what obligations researchers, sponsors, research institutions, governments and other stakeholders in the research process owe to participants and their communities. The authors of an article titled *Ethical Considerations Related to the Provision of Care and Treatment in Vaccine Trials*, point out that "[e]thical principles of beneficence and justice combined with international human rights norms and standards create certain obligations on researchers, sponsors and public health authorities…However, these obligations are poorly defined in practical terms; inconsistently understood or inadequately applied."[1] The case studies in this chapter are intended to stimulate thoughtful discussion of obligations in research, identifying who is responsible for providing those obligations and the process by which those obligations are discussed and negotiated. Although this discussion of obligations is pertinent to all research, the case studies here focus on international research in developing countries.

In addition to the article just cited – which provides a very good table of considerations regarding obligations relevant to good research governance – two recent guidance documents provide useful frameworks for thinking about these issues both in broad theoretical terms and in a very practical manner. Although they focus on HIV prevention trials, they may prove useful in other research contexts as well.

- Ethical Considerations in Biomedical HIV Prevention Trials. Geneva: UNAIDS and WHO, 2007. http://whqlibdoc.who.int/unaids/2007/9789291736256_eng.pdf (accessed 25 August 2008)

- Good Participatory Practices in the Conduct of Biomedical HIV Prevention Trials. Geneva: UNAIDS/AVAC, 2007. http://whqlibdoc.who.int/unaids/2007/9789291736348_eng.pdf (accessed 25 August 2008)

[1] Tarantola, op.cit., p. 23.

The topic of 'obligations in health research' is extremely broad and may contain too many wide-ranging issues for a short classroom or workshop discussion. As a facilitator, you may find that the discussion is of a higher quality with more analytical depth if very specific issues are examined systematically. You may, for example, wish to separate out a discussion of what participants and other stakeholders believe should be the obligations to participants and their families, from a discussion of the process by which those obligations are negotiated and who is charged with fulfilling them. The article by L. Belsky and H.S. Richardson titled *Medical Researchers' Ancillary Clinical Care Responsibilities*[1] provides an interesting framework which may be helpful for facilitating a discussion on obligations. The *Good Participatory Practices* document cited above addresses the process of discussing obligations. Facilitators may also want to be aware of the range of non-negotiable obligations placed on research by some national bodies, as well as by international guidelines.

The case studies in this chapter address questions of who is obligated and what their obligations are. This list is not exhaustive but should be seen as providing some initial ideas. Examples include obligations to research participants

- who are harmed as the result of research. Does it make a difference whether or not the healthcare system is accessible to the people who are research participants when determining the obligation to treat the harm?

- who experience a serious adverse event (and how is this defined?) Is pregnancy during a contraceptive trial a SAE?

- who are discovered by the researchers during enrolment screening to have a condition (HIV for example) other than the target disease Do researchers or sponsors have any obligation to provide care for such a condition or other benefits such as general health care, counselling, nutritional supplements, follow up care for short term or chronic conditions? What about for conditions that arise during the research? Does it matter whether they are related or unrelated to the intervention or disease being studied?

There may also be obligations to people who are not research participants, e.g. those who

- are directly negatively affected by any earnings loss or other harm to the participant

- live in close proximity to a participant receiving benefits and who may also be in need of those benefits (such as an older child in a poor household whose younger sibling is taking part in a study on the effects of nutritional supplements on young children's learning).

- need to be protected, based on information gained during research, such as when a researcher learns of abusive behaviour by a parent or drug abuse by a child. This also raises privacy and confidentiality issues that are examined in the next chapter.

- require someone to advocate for, or to give them, broad access to successful interventions.

Finally, is there an obligation to increase research and health literacy (knowledge and skill building)?

Chapter VII: Privacy and Confidentiality

The case studies in this chapter are designed to encourage students and workshop participants to explore the many dilemmas that confront researchers in their attempts to uphold confidentiality and to protect privacy. Facilitators may want to begin by introducing the idea that the value placed on confidentiality and privacy is not universal but varies by culture. Some cultures or communities are suspicious of the emphasis on privacy and confidentiality or would understand a completely different set of actions as manifestations of privacy and confidentiality. Recognizing that there are various understandings of what is meant by those terms, as well as the different cultural value placed on them, can help the student or workshop participant to think through the purposes, and the limitations, of confidentiality and privacy in the research context.

---

[1] Belsky L, Richardson HS. Medical Researchers' Ancillary Clinical Care Responsibilities. *British Medical Journal*, 2004;328:1494-1496.
http://dx.doi.org/10.1136/bmj.328.7454.1494 (accessed 25 August 2008)

Duties of privacy and confidentiality also have consequences for data protection, for who controls access to information, and for public health. This issue is explored in the article in the chapter reading list titled *Public Health and Data Protection: An Inevitable Collision or a Meeting of Minds?*[1] (The many issues raised by genomic research and data banks are not explored in the case studies but increasingly are becoming issues for researchers in international health research.) Issues related to the principles of confidentiality and privacy that facilitators may want to explore include:

- Whether there are there any limits to the expectation of confidentiality. If, in the course of research, a researcher learns of illegal, unethical or dangerous behaviour, should this be reported? Are there national or local laws which are applicable? What should happen if a consent form stating that all information will be kept confidential has been signed but it becomes clear that the participant poses a danger to him or herself, or to others? Should the informed consent form indicate that there are limits? What if reporting the illegal behaviour will likely result in the authorities (police or parents, for example) responding in a manner that the researcher thinks will be overly harsh? Some situations where the limits of confidentiality can be explored include:

    - researcher knowledge of child abuse

    - diagnosis of a contagious disease which could pose a public health threat

    - observational studies of dangerous or life-threatening behaviour to self or others involving a vulnerable person (an infant being fed with dirty water, a needle being reused in a health centre, a teenager who expresses a suicide plan)

    - illegal abortions resulting in post-abortion complications

    - focus group participants sharing information from the FG despite having been asked not to do so.

- How are confidentiality and privacy best achieved and maintained? What measures are in place and are these adequate?

    - When conducting research with a population who has disease that creates stigma, as is often the case with tuberculosis or HIV/AIDS, what extra precautions, if any, should be taken to ensure confidentiality (e.g. study data kept in a locked filing cabinet)?

    - Has adequate anonymisation (or other de-linking process) occurred for all data including samples stored for future use? Are all stakeholders aware of the need for confidentiality and how to maintain it? Who has legal rights to the data and for how long? When can the data be destroyed? How safe are electronic records?

Chapter VIII: Professional Ethics

The case studies in this chapter focus on two aspects of professional ethics: conflicts of interest and scientific misconduct.

A discussion of conflicts of interest – which arises when an investigator can obtain money or comparable personal benefits through behaviour that is not consistent with his or her professional obligations as a physician and/or scientist – can encompass a number of important topics:

- In some countries, a majority of faculty in medical schools have financial links to industries in their field.[2] What effect would this be expected to have on rules about conflicts of interest?

---

[1] Lawlor DA, Stone T. Public Health and Data Protection: An Inevitable Collision or Potential for a Meeting of Minds? *International Journal of Epidemiology*, 2001; 30:1221-1225.
http://ije.oxfordjournals.org/cgi/content/full/30/6/1221
(accessed 9 May 2008)

[2] Campbell EG et al., Institutional Academic-Industry Relationships. JAMA 2007; 298:15: 1779-1786.

- The trend toward commercially funded research and testing has been accompanied by a variety of financial incentives for investigators to recruit patients rapidly and to allow other ethically questionable practices such as "ghostwriting" (i.e. a scientist's agreement, that a paper actually written by a company employee can be published under the scientist's name). Some argue that these incentives stimulate innovation and the rapid translation of laboratory advances into therapeutic products. Critics argue that such arrangements threaten the integrity of scientists and of medical science.

- Are all conflicts of interest inherently wrong, or is it only wrong when someone who has a conflict of interest behaves wrongly?

- Which conflicts of interest are inconsistent with a professional being responsible for patient care? With being responsible for research design and conduct?

- What about conflicts that arise not from financial rewards but from an investigator's commitment to a particular set of ideas or theories? How do such conflicts differ from financial conflicts, for example, in the risks they raise for research participants, for the integrity of research, and in the means available to uncover and mitigate the conflicting interest?

- What evidence of conflict of interest should be routinely collected by research ethics committees? Is it their responsibility to ensure that the reports of conflicts of interest are complete and accurate, or should they rely on the investigator's integrity?

- What constitutes conflict of interest for a member of a research ethics committee? What precautions or remedies should be undertaken?

"Scientific misconduct" is the deliberate falsification of scientific data, or a distortion in the reporting of scientific data; it also encompasses similar violations of the internal norms of scientific investigation. While once regarded as unusual, these offences now appear to be more widespread and have been the target of investigations by governments, funding sources, universities, and journalists. Among the issues to explore in case-based discussions are:

- Are norms of scientific conduct – and, therefore, criteria for judging scientific misconduct – variable across regions and national boundaries? Or is science a single, global profession with common standards?

- What forms of scientific misconduct are the most serious? Which are the proper concern of research ethics committees?

- Who is responsible for identifying scientific misconduct (e.g. peers, staff, employers, journal editors, sponsors, government regulators)? If those deemed responsible do not take action, what are the responsibilities of others who learn of the misconduct, including research ethics committee members?

Additional resources for case based teaching

Fourtner, A.W., Fourtner CR. and Herreid CF. **"Case Teaching Notes for "Bad Blood:" A Case Study of the Tuskegee Syphilis Project"** University at Buffalo, state University of New York

http://ublib.buffalo.edu/libraries/projects/cases/blood_notes.html (accessed 2 May 2009)

Herriod CF. **Return to Mars – How Not to Teach a Case Study**

http://ublib.buffalo.edu/libraries/projects/cases/teaching/mars.html (accessed 2 May 2009)

Husock, H. **"Using a Teaching Case"**, Kennedy School of Government Case Program. Harvard University: 2000

http://www.ksgcase.harvard.edu/ (accessed 7 April 2009)

Pimple KD. **Using Case Studies in Teaching Research Ethics**

http://poynter.indiana.edu/tre/kdp-cases.pdf
(accessed 2 June 2009)

Waterman, MA., Stanley, EDA. "**Assessing Case Learning**"
Case Based Learning in Your Classes. Author copyright 2004

http://cstl-csm.semo.edu/waterman/CBL/
(accessed 2 June 2009)

The Case Studies

Chapter I

Defining "Research"

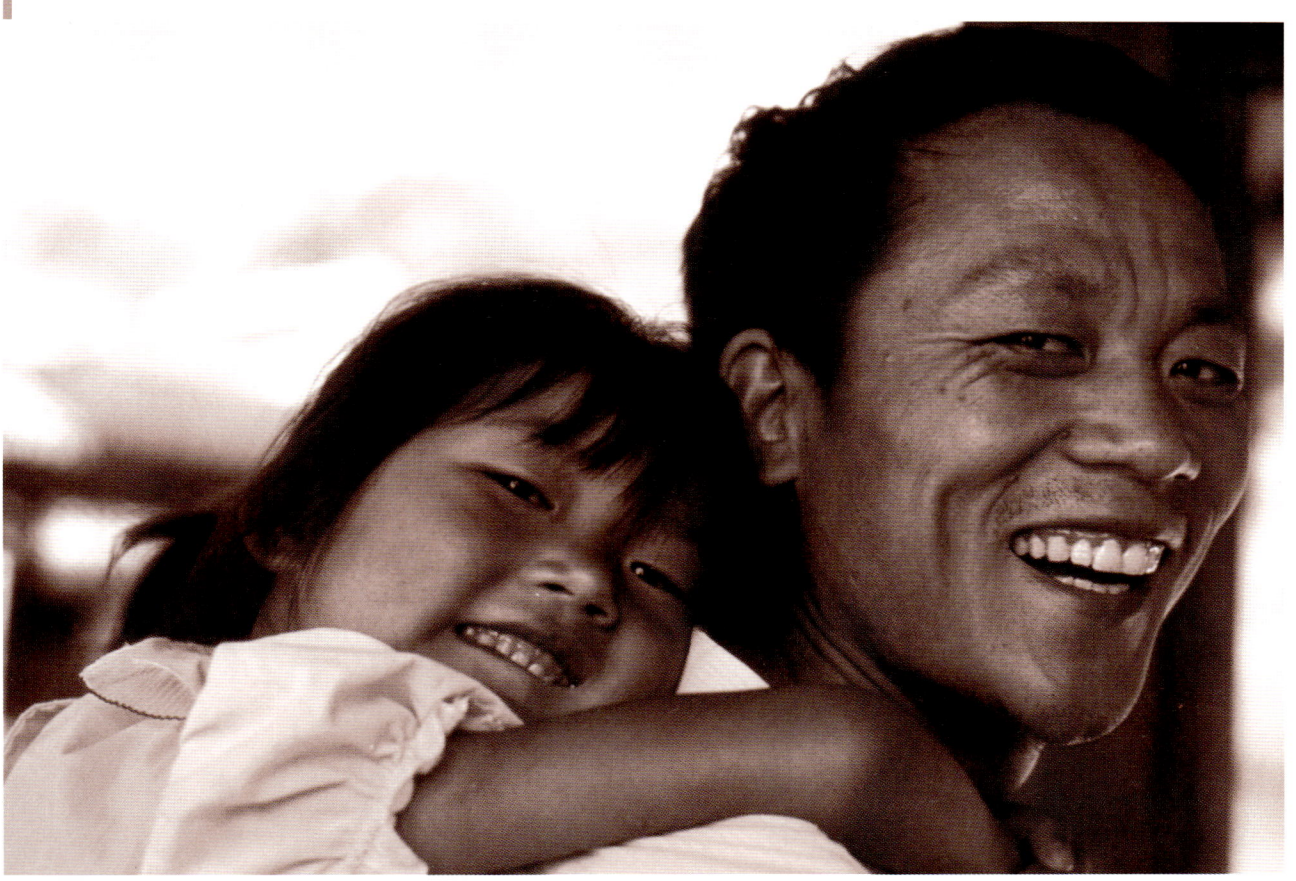

© WHO/Pierre Virot

Introduction: Chapter I

When must an ethics committee's approval be sought?

The need for a definition of 'research', for the purposes of ethical review, is closely related to a practical decision: what kinds of activities should be subject to review by a research ethics committee (REC)? But defining what is meant by 'research' involves matters of principle not just management. The case studies in this chapter explore the boundaries of research by examining what identifies research as distinct from medical treatment or from other activities involving the collection and analysis of data for surveillance, health impact assessment, and quality-improvement assessments. In turn, decisions can be made about which activities need to be reviewed and approved by a research ethics committee.

One way of thinking about health research with human beings could be that it includes any social science, biomedical or epidemiological activity that entails systematic collection or analysis of data with the intent to generate new knowledge, in which human beings

- are exposed to manipulation, intervention, observation, or other interaction with investigators either directly, or through alteration of their environment, or

- become individually identifiable through investigators' collection, preparation, or use of biological material or medical or other records.

Confusing uncertainty with research

Every time a physician treats a patient, even with a well-established therapy, an element of uncertainty arises: what results will the intervention produce in this instance, and, more particularly, will any unwanted side-effects or more serious harms occur? Physicians therefore sometimes say that every treatment amounts to an experiment, and that the element of experimentation becomes even more pronounced when, as frequently occurs, they vary routine medical regimens in small (and sometimes not so small) ways, trying to achieve better results than those produced by a standard approach. Describing such therapeutic interventions – whether they are a slight deviation from a standard treatment or whether they are highly innovative – as experiments does not violate ordinary usage, but for several reasons these interventions should not be confused with research.

The primary intent of research is knowledge production

In cases where research aims to test the effect of a new intervention, such as a drug or vaccine, the principal difference between treatment (whether standard or innovative) and research is that treatment is undertaken to benefit the particular patient while research is undertaken to produce new scientific knowledge. This difference in intent has not only operational consequences (in the way research interventions are designed and carried out so as to allow valid conclusions to be drawn) but also moral significance.

The people who agree to be participants in research might be fortunate and benefit directly from doing so, but *the production of knowledge – not benefits to participants – is the common factor in all health research*. Conversely, new knowledge may sometimes emerge from patient care, especially from an innovative therapy, but that does not change the initial intent, which is to benefit an individual patient. The people who conduct research might, of course, have additional motivations: a scientist might hope to achieve career success, or a research sponsor might expect to earn a profit from a new drug, but these ends depend (or should depend) on fulfilling the purpose of the study, which is to discover or validate a way to protect or restore health.

However, not all research is carried out to test new interventions or drugs, and not all research is with individual patients. Research often involves healthy volunteers, and in public health, involves whole communities or populations. As the awareness of the social determinants of health increases, so does the range of sociobehavioural and ethnographic research that is carried out on individuals and communities. Increasingly, governments are keen to collect a range of information from their populations (e.g. demographic and health surveys), and although some of these surveys might not be regarded as research, because their purpose is to guide policy rather than generate new knowledge, they often include research questions, which can blur the distinction between what is research and what is not.

Not letting the quest for knowledge override human welfare

The production of scientific knowledge does not relieve scientists – particularly those in the health professions – of other duties, including the obligation to protect the human beings who serve as research participants from avoidable harm or unjustified risks. Unfortunately, failures of scientists to honour this obligation have marred the history of research. The Nazi experiments on concentration camp prisoners during the Second World War are the most notorious instance, but other examples have occurred in many other countries both before and after the war crimes trial of the Nazi doctors in Nuremberg in 1947. In all these cases, the scientific mission (and possibly political zeal) so completely dominated the investigators' actions that they caused or allowed terrible harm to occur, in addition to exposing research participants to risk without their knowledge or consent.

In all biomedical and health research, the division between the interests of research participants and those of the researchers is important. This division, or conflict of mission, becomes particularly evident in clinical trials in which a physician assumes the role of investigator towards his or her patients, who then become simultaneously patients and research participants. Such "therapeutic research" serves as a reminder that when two activities (therapy and research) are combined it is easy to forget how divergent their objectives really are.

In other types of research, no explicit conflict of missions might exist since collection of data is the only immediate purpose, for example, samples and specimens collected for databanks, but research participants might agree to take part on the mistaken assumption that investigators from the health field always come with the potential to provide health care and access to health care (the so-called "therapeutic misconception"). Finally, research can cause other types of harm that might not be so obvious, but that could be more severe than the potential for physical harm associated with clinical research. For example, sociobehavioural research that explores sensitive information about participants' conduct, could allow the actions or responses of research participants to become known to others, and therefore could cause social or psychological harm. A second example is formative research, or research carried out before the conduct of full-blown large-scale clinical trials. Though often innocuous, formative research has the potential to cause harm or embarrassment to communities.

Managing the conflict between scientific and protective goals

How the potential conflict between scientific and therapeutic (or humanitarian) missions should be managed is the central question of research ethics. A rule requiring that the interests of human participants receive absolute priority and protection would prevent many harms to research participants, and many investigators insist on this standard. But taken literally, such a rule would preclude a large proportion of health research, including research that seems relatively uncontroversial. For example, to study an antiviral drug, healthy people might be exposed to a so-called viral challenge, in which they would be deliberately exposed to the virus before being given either the drug being tested or a placebo. Although such a study would clearly be unethical with a virus that is known to cause serious harm or death, might it not be acceptable to expose well-informed volunteers to a virus that could produce, at most, the symptoms of a moderate head cold?

Unless a rule is adopted that bars all research with the potential to jeopardize participants' well-being, then some ethical guidance is needed to decide what research should and should not be undertaken. At one time, this judgment was left solely in the hands of researchers, guided by their own conscience and the advice and oversight of their peers. In passing judgment on the Nazi doctors, the court articulated a set of principles for ethically permissible research with human beings (which came to be known as the Nuremberg Code[1]); the first principle is that the consent of any participant is absolutely essential. This means that the decision about whether to proceed with research should depend on participants giving informed consent to participate in a study that is designed by a researcher according to additional ethical standards, such as the minimization of harm to participants and an appropriate balance of potential benefits and harms.

The mandate and limitations of research ethics committees (RECS)

Having found – through the ethical failings of several prominent medical studies[2]– that unjustifiable research could not be prevented if decisions were left solely to investigators and participants, research funders and regulators now insist that an independent committee, constituted for this purpose, oversees the management and balancing of risks and benefits to research participants and research communities. Such committees are variously called Research Ethics Committees (RECs), human subject protection committees, institutional review boards (IRBs), or independent ethics committees, but in this book, they are referred to as RECs. The mandate of RECs does not rest solely on participants in health research being exposed to risk; rather, research must undergo prior review by a REC because it involves a conflict of missions for the medical scientists or for the sponsors.

One consequence of mandating RECs to deal only with activities that involve a conflict between scientific and therapeutic missions, is that RECs are then clearly not an all-purpose mechanism to prevent wrong-doing in hospitals and research institutions. For example, it is possible that individual therapeutic innovations may seriously injure or cause the deaths of more patients than do research studies. But a research ethics committee is limited to overseeing interventions that involve the conflict between the scientific and the therapeutic (or humanitarian) mission; it is not constituted to oversee medical interventions, even though they may be high risk. If an innovative therapy is re-defined as research in order to ensure both oversight and the broadest benefits from utilizing the intervention, and if it follows the standards demanded by scientific research (protocol development, scientific review by peers), then a REC would be appropriate. Otherwise, another committee or mechanism should deal with the issues that arise from potentially risky innovative therapies.

Finally, two related points need to be made. First, there are times when a REC may choose to waive a review *even if the activity is research*, and second, not all conflicts of missions involve research and require REC oversight.

As to the first, a REC may waive ethical oversight of the research because the proposed research study *clearly* poses no risk for participants, as, for example, with an anonymous telephone survey. It is, however, not always easy to determine risk; for example, certain types of health-related social science research may have been considered low risk in the past but new knowledge has raised awareness that even questionnaires and surveys may put participants at risk for repercussions.

---

[1] Nuremberg Code. In: Trials of War Criminals Before the Nuremberg Military Tribunals Under Control Council Law No. 10, Vol. 2, Nuremberg, October 1946-April 1949. Permissible Medical Experiments on Human Subjects. Washington: United States Government Printing Office (2), 1949:181-182.
http://www.hhs.gov/ohrp/references/nurcode.htm (accessed 28 August 2008)

[2] See, for example, Beecher HK, Ethics and Clinical Research. *The New England Journal of Medicine*, 1966, 274: 1354-1360.

Another example of assumed low risk research is operations research on health care systems, their structures, and their environments which aims to analyse key issues, problems, and challenges in order to improve delivery of health care. Although operations research might be carried out on health care providers, it often involves the people who receive health care and is not always as low risk as it is typically assumed to be. For example, if operations research were undertaken to determine whether a particular health system had the capacity to administer a rapid diagnostic test for an infectious disease, the communities in the study would probably receive better care and treatment for that disease during the study period, resulting in temporary or longer term inequities within the health system. Similarly, studies carried out to assess the efficacy of new management guidelines or treatment schedules could benefit patients, but could also uncover inefficiencies in the system for which individuals were responsible. In this instance, the research may not be low risk for those responsible for poor decisions. How could the researchers ensure that such knowledge would not harm the professional careers of people who took part as research participants?

As to the second point, RECs might not have jurisdiction over non-research activities such as public health surveillance or certain evaluation activities, even though they involve a conflict of missions. For example, in routine public health surveillance of infectious diseases, one goal is to maintain the well-being of individuals under observation, and another is to prevent the spread of disease to the general population. Yet resolving the potential conflict between benefit to the individual and the good of the population relies on mechanisms other than RECs. These mechanisms could include either laws that authorize officials to act in the interest of public health, even without informed consent if that would jeopardize public health objectives, or health officials' accountability to the public through various mechanisms, including, perhaps, a body to provide prior review of the surveillance to ensure that public health authorities strike the right balance between individual and group interests. Although most RECs operate outside these processes, in some instances a research question is appended to a public health activity that is still in progress. Who should provide ethical oversight in such situations often falls into a grey area, creating a risk that research activities that should be submitted to RECs go un-reviewed.

Suggested readings

Centers for Disease Control and Prevention. Guidelines for Defining Public Health Research and Public Health Non-Research. Revised October 4, 1999. Atlanta, GA, USA: CDC, 1999.

This document "sets forth CDC guidelines on the definition of public health research conducted by CDC staff irrespective of the funding source (i.e. provided by CDC or by another entity). Under Federal regulations (45 CFR 46), the final determination of what is research and whether the Federal regulations are applicable lies with CDC and, ultimately, with the Office for Protection from Research Risks (OPRR) [now the Office for Human Research Protections or 'OHRP']." The guidance is intended for use by state and local health departments and other institutions that conduct collaborative research with CDC staff or that are recipients of CDC funds.

http://www.cdc.gov/od/science/regs/hrpp/researchDefinition.htm (accessed 9 May 2008)

Wade DT. Ethics, Audit, and Research: All Shades of Grey. *British Medical Journal*, 2005, 330: 468-471.

"All research studies have to be scrutinized by an ethics committee [...] but most ethics committees specifically exclude audit studies from their remit. Similarly, journal editors and funding agencies will require evidence of ethical review before accepting research for publication or funding but do not require this for audit studies. Consequently, the distinction between audit and research can have important implications, and the temptation to label research as audit is considerable." This article reviews the difficult distinction between audit and research, and includes four illustrative case studies which readers are invited to analyze and respond to.

http://dx.doi.org/10.1136/bmj.330.7489.468
(accessed 25 August 2008)

Case 1

SARS and airplane passengers

In Country X, public health responsibilities are lodged in a national centre which carries out routine surveillance of diseases in association with local health agencies, and disseminates information as an aid to disease control and prevention. In March 2003, during the worldwide outbreak of a new human pathogen labelled severe acute respiratory syndrome (SARS), the national centre aimed to systematically identify both people with potential cases of SARS and any individuals who had been within contact range of those people. Since the disease originated outside the country, concern centred on people who arrived from parts of the world where SARS cases had occurred.

As part of these activities, officials of the centre focused on potential SARS cases arising from casual contact between airline passengers or crew members. If an individual who was suspected or known to be infected with SARS (an "index case") gave a history of having recently flown into the country, the centre would first obtain the flight manifest from the airline.[1] Then the centre would call on local public health agencies to locate people listed on the flight manifest who might have been exposed to the index case of SARS.

The process of obtaining flight manifests and locating named individuals often caused a delay of 3-4 weeks between the time the centre suspected a potential exposure and when an investigation could take place. Nevertheless, the centre's officials requested that local public health agents ask physicians to draw blood samples and obtain medical histories of apparently healthy, unaffected air travellers who were on the plane with the index case. As administrative delays mounted, the time to test the blood of asymptomatic individuals would have surpassed the likely incubation period for SARS; thus, the tests could at most have revealed that they might have been exposed.[2] Nonetheless, the national centre wanted this data because so little was known about SARS, how it was transmitted, whether some people were more or less susceptible to it, and how it affected different individuals.

Questions

1 Were the data collected for surveillance, for disease prevention or for research?

2 Should approval have been obtained from a research ethics committee? Should informed consent forms have been required?

Adapted and included with permission from: Hodge J, Gostin L. Public Health Practice vs. Research: Report for Public Health Practitioners Including Cases and Guidance for Making Distinctions. Atlanta, GA, USA, Council of State and Territorial Epidemiologists, 2004.
www.cste.org/pdffiles/newpdffiles/CSTEPHRes RptHodgeFinal.5.24.04.pdf, (accessed 26 March 2008)

---

[1] A flight manifest is a list of passengers and crew of an aircraft which is compiled before departure and is based on flight check-in information.

[2] WHO estimates the maximum incubation period to be 10 days.

Case 2

Evaluating sexual health and family planning programmes

The Institute for Family and Youth has a contract with a bilateral funding agency to implement family planning and sexually transmitted infections (STI) and HIV prevention programmes in developing countries. The funding is conditional on inclusion of an evaluation component. Through its "Healthy Ideas!" programme, the Institute has recently established three public health prevention projects in developing countries:

- An HIV testing and counselling programme for adolescents with sites in one country in each of three regions (eastern Europe, sub-Saharan Africa, and South-East Asia) which will be evaluated using questionnaire surveys of adolescents over a 3-year period to investigate frequency and types of drug use, sexual activity, and sexual preference.

- The second project will provide prenatal care to a poor, urban community located in a country where HIV infection is still highly stigmatizing. The evaluation component will examine the frequency of partner-notification among married and unmarried women whom the clinic diagnoses as HIV-positive.

- The third is a condom education project which will be located in a South American city with rapidly rising incidences of STIs and HIV. It has been modelled after a "100% condom use" programme found to be effective in South-East Asia, in which graduated sanctions are imposed on brothel owners based on the rate of STIs found among female sex workers in brothels. Ultimately, the brothel runs the risk of closure if sex workers repeatedly get STIs. An evaluation is planned to assess the feasibility of implementing the condom programme.

The Institute for Family and Youth says these projects do not need clearance from a research ethics committee because the activities are low risk, do not test an intervention, and are "operations research," not biomedical research. The head of evaluations at the Institute cites "human subjects research" regulations in the United States of America under which she believes ongoing evaluations of actual interventions are not subject to ethical review. She also stresses that the findings of the evaluations will be used to help design better public health programmes for the other sites where the Institute runs disease prevention programmes.

Questions

1. Are any of these projects research studies? Explain why or why not.

2. What distinguishes research from ongoing evaluations of public health interventions?

3. Do these activities require any ethical oversight?

4. The Institute for Family and Youth says that these projects are low risk. Discuss what is meant by "low risk" in the context of an ethics review? Does the level of risk affect whether or not it needs to be reviewed?

Adapted from "What is Research" contributed by Joan Atkinson and Nancy Kass, Johns Hopkins Bloomberg School of Public Health and Johns Hopkins Berman Institute of Bioethics.

Case 3

A treatment for central nervous system conditions

Dr W is a neurosurgeon in a hospital in one of Asia's major metropolitan centres. He earned his medical degree in that city and then studied in the United States of America before returning to practise in his own country. Over the past 3 years, Dr W has treated more than 500 patients with central nervous system (CNS) conditions – including amyotrophic lateral sclerosis (ALS, also known as Lou Gehrig's disease), Parkinson's disease, stroke, paraplegia, and tetraplegia – by injecting these patients' brains or spinal cords with olfactory stem cells harvested from the noses of aborted fetuses. Dr W is convinced that this intervention, which he describes to patients as an "innovative therapy," is effective, and he has declined to conduct a controlled clinical trial of this method.

Cell transplantation experiments have been undertaken for several decades and continue to be pursued in several countries. Dr W's method is unique, however, because he uses olfactory ensheathing cells from fetuses aborted at 16 weeks. The women who agree to allow the cell harvesting of their aborted fetuses all provide consent and do not receive payment or other compensation. Using a hypodermic syringe, Dr W transplants the culled cells into paralysed patients above and below the damaged area of the spinal cord; ALS patients receive the injections directly into the atrophied area of the frontal lobe of the brain, through a small hole drilled in the skull (a burr hole).

Despite having only an incomplete explanation of how the injections produce their results, Dr W is convinced by his patients' outcomes that the method works. Both lay and medical publications have reported the positive results of the treatment, and Dr W recently submitted an article to a local journal describing his success. Many of his current patients come from other countries to receive his treatment.

Long-term follow-up data on Dr W's work remains preliminary. However, patients – particularly those who have spinal injuries – whom he has contacted by e-mail several months after their operations have reported continued progress. The only adverse effect noted had been pain that accompanied restoration of feeling in some patients. Dr W claims that the surgery stabilizes the condition in about 50% of his patients, and that it causes an improvement in the quality of life (QOL) in about 70% of patients. His estimates are derived from videos he has taken of patients before and after surgery, as well as a survey he conducted of 142 patients, using criteria for function assessment established by a North American spinal injury association.

Dr W's supporters, including the chair of a spinal neurosurgery programme at a leading North American university, have urged him to conduct double-blind trials to meet the scientific standards of developed countries. Since no recognized treatments can reverse the CNS conditions that his patients have, the intervention given to the control group in a double-blind study would be an injection of an inert fluid instead of the stem cells or "sham surgery" on the skull or spine (surgery to drill a hole and then close up the site, without putting in any cells). Research trials of this type have been used previously for other cellular treatments for neurological diseases, but Dr W refuses to do this, asserting that such studies would be unethical. "Even if the whole world refuses to believe me, I would not do a control test," he says. "These patients are already suffering. If we open them up just for a placebo test, it will only do them harm. We would be doing it for ourselves not for the patient."

Questions

1. Is Dr W providing innovative therapy; conducting an experiment; or carrying out medical research? How are these different, generally or in this case?

2. Would it be unethical to conduct a placebo-controlled trial, as Dr W maintains?

3. How might Dr W demonstrate that this method is effective (other than by conducting a controlled clinical trial)? Is there an international standard for determining effectiveness?

4. In a hospital setting, whose responsibility is it to monitor the activities of physicians? In general, whose responsibility is it to monitor activities of physicians?

Case 4

Documenting the health conditions of an indigenous community

The farmers and forest workers of a largely rural district of South America have recently renewed contacts with an isolated indigenous community in order to gain access to their natural resources. The public health agency fears that this interaction will cause higher incidences of infectious diseases and possibly mortality in the indigenous people. The agency, therefore, invites a university research team to conduct an exploratory study to document the health conditions of this indigenous community. Financial resources are made available but are conditional upon all expenditures being committed by the end of the financial year – that is within a period of 3 months.

The research team accepts the challenge and develops a research study based on both a demographic survey (of every fifth household) and a clinical examination of research participants that includes taking blood samples for haematological, biochemical, and immunological tests. In addition, the investigators consider this a timely opportunity to undertake genetic characterization of this population, and include an analysis for genetic markers. As the community lacks residential addresses, the investigators propose to establish a photographic database to facilitate follow-up with individual participants.

After reviewing the protocol, the research ethics committee notes two major concerns: first, the researchers have not provided an adequate justification for blood sampling and, second, safeguards to protect participant confidentiality are lacking.

The investigators acknowledge the concerns of the research ethics committee, and promise to contact the public health agency to indicate a possible delay in starting the research. At the same time, however, the investigators feel themselves to be under pressure due to a tight timetable within the university, local preliminary plans, transportation arrangements, mobilization of the study team, and not least, their great motivation for the project. They reason that ethics approval was required only for blood collection and not for the collection of the demographic data. They decide to postpone the clinical examinations and blood collection until the protocol is revised and approved, but, meanwhile, to visit the community and move ahead with the survey research and photographic database. In fact, the investigators view this as an opportune time to begin to build trusting relationships within the community, and therefore to facilitate the consent for blood sampling once the approval of the committee has been gained.

Three days after beginning the survey, a 5 year-old child from one of the households selected for the survey comes down with meningitis. Members of the community blame the investigators, claiming that the photographs were being used by the local farmers to harm the tribe through witchcraft.

Questions

1. Were the investigators correct in their assumption that ethics approval is not required for the collection of demographic profiles? Why or why not?

2. Was what the researchers did "scientific misconduct"?

3. What are the special ethical concerns when dealing with minority or ethnically isolated communities? What safeguards might the ethics committee be referring to?

4. How might collection of blood samples for genetic characterization be harmful to this population?

5. What procedures can be put in place to ensure that this research brings benefit to this population?

6. How could the incident relating to the 5 year-old child have been averted? What, if any, are the investigators' obligations towards any child who becomes ill during the course of the study?

Adapted from a case study contributed by Dr Dirce Guilhem and Dr Fabio Zicker.

Chapter II

Issues in Study Design

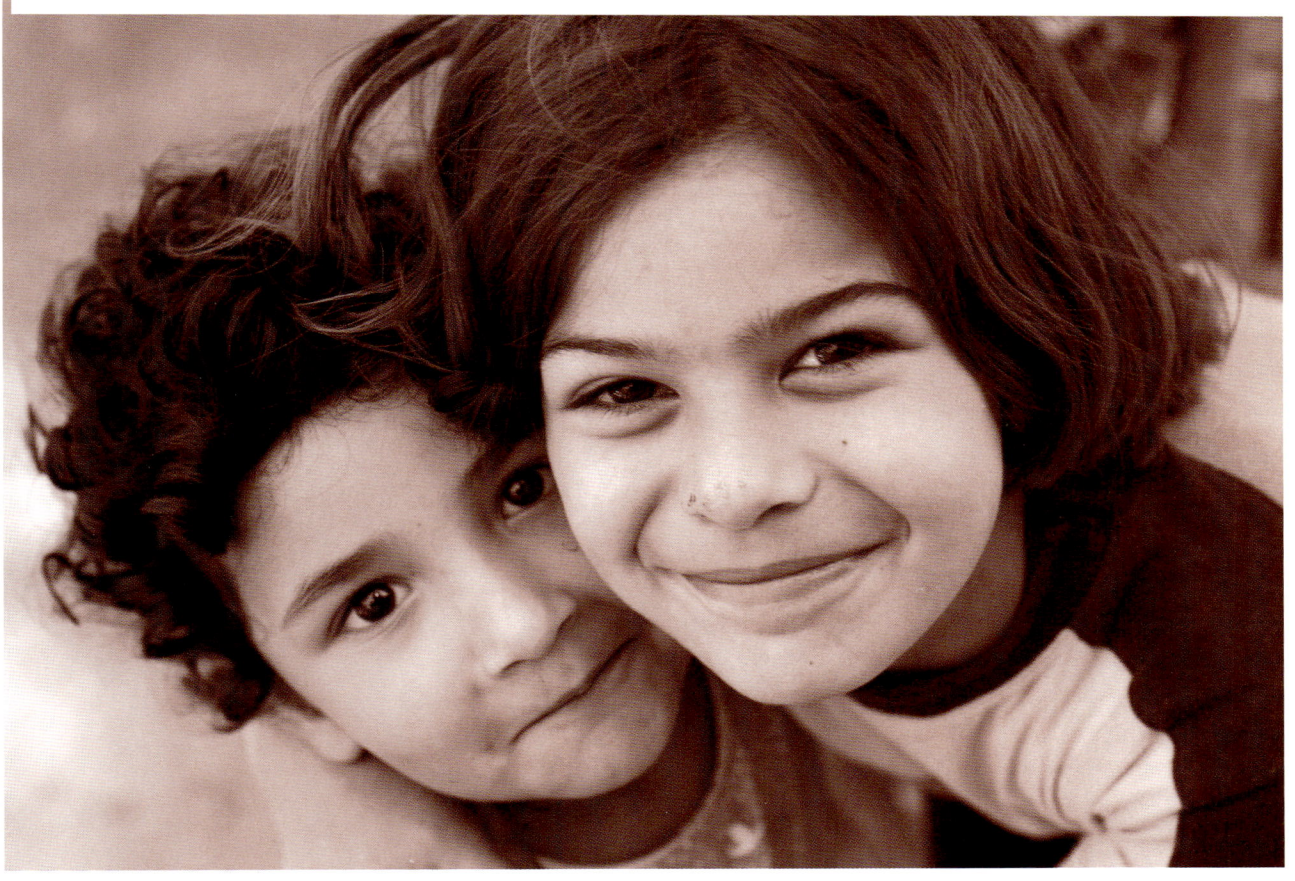

© WHO/Christopher Black

Introduction: Chapter II

Designing scientifically (and ethically) sound studies

One of the most contentious issues in research ethics is whether or not research ethics committees (RECs) should assess the scientific adequacy of the research protocols they review. RECs typically have this responsibility (although there may also be a scientific review committee constituted to do this) but the way that they do it is often harshly criticized by investigators. Division of this issue into two separate questions could therefore be useful:

- Is it a matter of ethical concern how well a research project is designed in scientific terms?
- Is the REC the right body to judge the scientific merits of a project's design?

Connecting scientific design to ethics

Exposure of research participants to physical or social harm, discomfort, or even inconvenience can be justified only when there is good reason to anticipate some compensating benefit to society (i.e. to the body of scientific knowledge or the well-being of future patients or society at large) and perhaps to the participants as well. A study with a design so flawed that nothing can be learned from it ought therefore not to be undertaken. In a phrase, bad science is bad ethics.

However, having a scientifically appropriate design is not enough to determine that a study meets ethical requirements. Scientists in some of the most brutal and inhumane experiments have pointed to scientific necessity to justify their research. Yet if they were correct in maintaining that the information they sought could not have been obtained without exposing human beings to inhumane conditions, *the conclusion that they should have reached* (but did not) was that it was morally wrong to conduct the research, and therefore the knowledge should have remained beyond reach. (This conclusion itself raises an ethical dilemma for subsequent researchers: is it ever ethically acceptable to rely on, or cite, studies which are apparently scientifically valid but whose results were obtained unethically, given that such results are otherwise unavailable from other, ethically acceptable sources?)

A more common issue is whether a scientifically appropriate design raises ethical concerns even though it does not obviously violate ethical (and perhaps human rights) norms. For example, a study's design might be satisfactory, or even optimal, in scientific terms but might impose a burden on research participants that could be avoided or reduced by a different design. If the alternative design is capable of producing results that are scientifically equivalent, then this alternative design, which lessens the risks to the research participants is ethically mandated. But suppose that the alternative design involves a reduction in the probable scientific value of the research? For example, one study design might be able to provide data that would conclusively confirm (or disprove) a research hypothesis, while an alternative design that would impose fewer burdens on research participants is likely to produce less definitive evidence. What if such less definitive scientific evidence is not good enough to allow a disease to be diagnosed or treated with certainty? What if the disease under consideration can cause death if not diagnosed or treated? Does one's conclusion change if the disease is only mildly incapacitating but not crippling or fatal? What if this disease kills children and not adults? As this example makes clear, once one accepts that scientific design can raise ethical issues, one might have to balance values from these competing realms.

Who should assess the science in the context of ethics review?

The second question – who should assess the scientific design of a research project? – has three facets. The first is a purely scientific assessment: can the design produce the results being sought, that is, is it "good science"? The second is an evaluation of the design in ethical terms: does it involve methods that are inherently unethical, and could its results be produced equally well by a design that exposed participants to less harm? The third is a decision about whether the results that the study could produce are worth the burden or risk to participants because they are better in scientific terms by a margin that is sufficiently greater than the results that could be expected from a less burdensome or risky design. There can be little doubt that the second and third tasks are central to the responsibilities of RECs in reviewing research proposals. Whether the REC also has the mandate for the first task is more a practical question than a matter of moral principle. An institution that has experience with peer review and supervision could provide independent scientific reviews of proposed scientific studies by bodies with greater expertise than its REC could hope to muster. Further, RECs that undertake this function without sufficient expertise might seek to block or alter proposed studies for the wrong reasons. If institutional resources permit separate scientific and ethical reviews, a division of labour thus has some merit.

Where resources are more constrained, as they often are in developing countries, institutions might have to count on the REC to assess protocols both scientifically and ethically. And even if resources are not at issue, a member of a REC who finds a major flaw in a study's design cannot in good conscience vote to approve it until the problem has been remedied. To ensure that RECs do as thorough a job as possible, they should usually include members who have appropriate backgrounds in research design or be able to consult or co-opt special advisors as needed.

Particular design issues: placebos

Probably the most widely debated ethical aspect of research design is the use of "placebo controls". These are participants who receive – in place of the intervention given to the "active" or "treatment" group – a substance which they accept as a medicine or therapy, but which actually does not contain an active medication or known therapeutic quality (a placebo). If study participants are randomly assigned to receive either the active treatment or the placebo, so that there is no other systematic difference between the groups, then outcomes in the active group that differ significantly from those in the control group (both benefits and harms) can be attributed to the active treatment.

Upon initial reflection, to offer a new 'treatment' to one group of people while apparently doing nothing for another might seem to be inherently unfair. But the rationale for testing out a new treatment on human beings in a trial is to provide proof one way or the other. Therefore the new treatment is actually something with unproven effects – bad as well as good. Whatever the hopes and expectations of the investigators (and research participants) might be (e.g. that an experimental drug will prove effective and will be free of serious adverse effects), the reality is that a new intervention's effectiveness has not been proven until the trial has been done. Until this has happened, any decision to use the intervention in patients is based on a prediction or hope of a good outcome, rather than on scientific evidence. (This is, of course, true of a great many – probably still the large majority – of treatments in routine clinical use that have never been scientifically tested.) Such a situation, in which an unbiased expert has a genuine uncertainty about whether the new treatment is better than nothing (a placebo) is called "clinical equipoise".[1]

The burden of justification for using a placebo is highest when an effective treatment already exists for the same condition because a new treatment could in theory be tested by giving the control group the existing treatment rather than a placebo. According to the *International Ethical Guidelines for Biomedical Research Involving Human Subjects* developed by the Council for International Organizations of Medical Sciences (CIOMS), "As a general rule, research subjects in the control group of a trial of a diagnostic, therapeutic, or preventive intervention should receive an established effective intervention.

---

[1] Although it might seem surprising that a new drug or other intervention would get to the point of being tested in human beings without a lot of preliminary evidence from laboratory and animal studies to show that it is effective, the annals of research are replete with studies of interventions which were strongly endorsed by physicians and drug companies and yet which were shown in controlled trials to be either ineffective, harmful, or both.

In some circumstances it may be ethically acceptable to use an alternative comparator, such as placebo or 'no treatment'".[1] Article 29 of the *Declaration of Helsinki* cautions against the use of a placebo, and recommends its use only in very select situations.[2] However, placebos are favoured by different groups for diverse reasons:

- Some research methodologists doubt the value of so-called head-to-head trials of new and existing treatments because evaluating the results is problematic.

- Some trial sponsors might favour placebo designs because they only have to demonstrate that their new product is safe and effective (i.e. better than nothing), rather than having to demonstrate that it is better than products that are already approved and in use.

- Placebo controls are most likely to raise ethical concerns when treatment options for the condition being studied are not available or accessible in the country in which the study is taking place. In such a situation, is it justifiable to use a placebo to test new drugs on the grounds that the existing treatment in that country is "no treatment"? This is linked to another ethical issue – is it justifiable to test a new drug, knowing that if it were found to be effective, it would not be available to the population or country in which it was first tested, because of its expense?

One way to avoid the dilemma is to limit placebo-controlled designs to studies in which there is genuine equipoise, that is, when there is no basis for differentiating the estimated net benefit for the active and placebo groups.[3] A physician-scientist who randomizes patient-participants between the active and control groups can then clearly affirm that the well-being of the patient has not been compromised for the sake of science.[4] Some commentators, however, insist that such equipoise is rare, and therefore would seldom allow placebo-controlled trials, while some take an even stronger position, arguing that in many clinical trials, if the facts were viewed dispassionately, rather than by people who are already convinced of the benefits of a new treatment, genuine equipoise would not exist at all. Other critics maintain that although genuine equipoise is relatively uncommon, this should not stand in the way of a placebo-controlled design if it is scientifically necessary. The latter position, however, requires giving up the claim that the investigators never compromise the well-being of participants for the sake of science.

In many instances, investigators have a choice: they can avoid placebo-controlled designs if they are willing to make certain compromises in terms of cost, time, and resources. Compared with some alternative study designs, placebo-controlled trials can be faster, cheaper, and need fewer participants to achieve a given level of certainty about the research hypothesis. A pharmaceutical company that is concerned with costs and with the need to bring products to the market quickly might be attracted by placebo designs for these reasons; likewise, a physician-investigator who wants to expose the smallest number of patients as possible to the risks inherent in a trial might also favour a placebo design. A REC must decide whether these advantages justify the decision to create a placebo-controlled arm in the study.

[1] Council for International Organizations of Medical Sciences (CIOMS). International Ethical Guidelines for Biomedical Research Involving Human Subjects. Geneva, Switzerland: Council for International Organizations of Medical Sciences (CIOMS), 2002. http://www.cioms.ch (accessed 9 May 2008)

[2] World Medical Association. *Declaration of Helsinki: Ethical Principles for Medical Research Involving Human Subjects.* Helsinki, Finland: WMA, 1964. Latest revised and updated version 2008. http://www.wma.net/e/policy/b3.htm (accessed 5 June 2009)

[3] Equipoise can be defined as a state of genuine uncertainty on the part of the expert medical community regarding the comparative therapeutic merits of each arm in a trial.

[4] What happens, however, when those assigned to one group *seem* to be more fortunate than the others?

Particular design issues: misleading studies

Tasked by current ethical guidelines to test new drugs against current effective therapies, pharmaceutical firms will often design trials in a manner that ensures that their product will test well. This can be achieved by planning inadequate blinding, by proposing the wrong analysis, or by using the comparator drug incorrectly or in ineffective dosages. These so-called Pollyanna designs are fraudulent exercises in marketing rather than science. What decision should a REC make if the submitted protocols seem to be otherwise ethically adequate? Only a narrow view of the REC role would confine its attention to the effects of the trial on its participants, ignoring such broader ethical issues of scientific design.

Particular design issues: observing natural experiments

Protecting the well-being of participants – a central concern of research ethics – has an important role in the evaluation of investigators' responsibility in so-called natural experiments. Although ethical scruples prevent investigators from placing participants at risk for very serious diseases, on occasion an opportunity will arise to study what happens when such a risk occurs without their interference. Suppose a group of people living in a highland area who lack immunity to malaria migrate to the lowlands where malaria is endemic. Investigators might wish to monitor their experience and to try out certain interventions under these circumstances. Is this study design morally acceptable, or should the investigators use all available existing means to protect this population from malaria, even if doing so would make the study impossible?

Another case: two groups of practitioners in a single medical group favour different treatments for a serious medical condition. The practitioner-investigators propose to compare outcomes without informing patients that they are participating in a comparison trial. Since each strongly favours one of the treatments over the other, they believe that equipoise does not exist. The investigators believe that what they view as inferior care is the result of the patients' choice of doctor and is not the investigators' responsibility. Is this a clever use of an available opportunity to obtain comparative data that might otherwise require an unethical experiment (involving random assignment in the absence of equipoise), or do the investigators have an obligation to inform their patients about the study and about their own views of the two treatments?

Particular design issues: observing practices in communities or health systems

Ethical issues that could go unnoticed unless particular attention is paid can occur in the design of observational studies. Many social scientists observe people as a they carry out their daily tasks and, based on the data collected, will come up with solutions on how health care could be delivered better. For example, a study that observes the way in which adolescents are provided with advice on reproductive health issues could recommend provision of more youth-friendly services or recruitment of younger staff to improve interaction between staff and clients. However the study data might actually show that particular health care providers are rude, do not do their jobs adequately, or provide some clients with the wrong advice. Should such scenarios be thought of and addressed in the protocol? Is it ethical to protect those who are not doing their jobs? Is it the role of the investigator to address what might be health systems problems or at best the negligent behaviour of an individual? How does the REC address such issues?

Issues of fairness, access, and relevance

The appropriateness and validity of the scientific design are not the only ethical issues that need to be considered by an investigator in planning a study or by a REC in reviewing it. Two other issues are also of central importance, although they are frequently overlooked. The first is something that should concern RECs whenever they scrutinize research projects – namely, are the selection criteria for participants fair? Why was a particular population chosen (say, patients at a public clinic rather than those who visit private physicians' offices), and within that population, are the bases for including and excluding individuals not only scientifically sound but also free of social bias? From the standpoint of justice, the research should not impose the risks and burdens inherent in research on an arbitrarily selected subset of people, particularly those who are least able to avoid such an imposition. Research studies are, for example, routinely carried out in communities with low socioeconomic status. Similarly, when a research team requests the nurses or students of their institution to enrol, the RECs need to be vigilant to the issue of possible coercion. On the other hand, in the past, women (especially those in the reproductive age group) and children were routinely excluded from research studies, mainly because they were considered to be vulnerable and it was assumed that protection meant excluding them from studies. Since treatments have therefore had to be extrapolated from studies done on men, relatively little is now known about the safety and efficacy of such treatments for women and children, rendering their care a sort of uncontrolled experiment.[1]

The second ethical issue involving study design that goes beyond scientific soundness relates to the purpose of the research. The logic of health research is that it is better to develop sound knowledge about the effects of interventions through controlled studies that expose a few people to harm (or a lack of benefit) than to introduce innovations without such knowledge and potentially expose the whole population to such risks. Particularly when research involves the development of therapies, one compensation to participants for taking part in a clinical trial is that they may potentially benefit in a direct way from participating (although such benefit is never the primary purpose or justification of the research, which is instead to produce scientific knowledge). But the framework for this participation is that the real benefit will come once the trial is completed, and the intervention is known to be safe and useful. For this logic to apply, the participants must be drawn from a group of people who stand some realistic change of enjoying that ultimate benefit, namely, having access to the fruits of the research.

This issue is of particular salience in international research for another reason. When, for example, a sponsor from a developed country comes to a developing country to run a clinical trial on a new drug, if the drug will be exclusively (or even, primarily) available to patients in developed countries after the trial, it needs to be asked whether it is appropriate to conduct the study in the developing country. Ethical guidance on international collaborative research insists that to be ethical, research must be relevant to the health needs of the country in which it is done. The guidance documents tend to be less clear, however, about how this is to be ensured. Can – and should – this question be confronted by RECs? Or do such questions need to be addressed at a higher level, by people in governmental ministries who are charged with health, research, and international affairs, when they decide whether to permit the foreign research organization to come into the country to run a clinical trial? Some commentators have suggested that this matter can best be addressed through prior agreements between trial sponsors and the host government. From an ethical standpoint, what objectives are appropriate in such negotiations? Should the host government flatly refuse to allow research that does not aim to develop means of prevention and treatment for the major health burdens that affect its population, or can the government legitimately allow its population to volunteer to be test participants (some would say "human guinea pigs"), even if the research will not provide the country with general access to the health intervention being tested? What if the trial sponsor offers to compensate the country by providing other benefits that the government believes would be of even greater value?

---

[1] The recent UNAIDS/WHO Biomedical HIV Prevention Trial Guidelines recommend the inclusion of women and children in trials and discuss how this can be done ethically. See UNAIDS/WHO. Ethical Considerations in Biomedical HIV Prevention Trials – UNAIDS/WHO guidance document. Geneva, Switzerland: Joint United Nations Programme on HIV/AIDS (UNAIDS) and the World Health Organization, 2007.
http://whqlibdoc.who.int/unaids/2007/9789291736256_eng.pdf
(accessed 25 August 2008)

The REC's role in assessing the ethics (including the science) of research designs

The first requirement for a REC assessing a research design involving human participants is to ensure that the committee fully comprehends the design of the protocol: what information the study seeks to gain, how it proposes to do this, and what effect its choice of design has on participants relative to alternative designs. If the design imposes risks or other burdens on participants that are not compensated by potential benefits, the REC can seek to determine whether comparable information could be obtained by the use of a different design that would reduce the burden or restrict the number of people who are exposed to risk. Trade-offs between the scientific merit of a design and the well-being of participants defy easy categorization and, as with many other issues within the REC's purview, are matters of moral judgment rather than compliance with checklists. If the burden on participants cannot be reduced without undermining the scientific integrity of the study, the committee must weigh this burden against the potential benefit to society. Of course, in some situations the REC might consider the burden to be so great that no amount of societal benefit can justify the study. The REC must also ensure that the selection of participants is equitable. Whether participants have genuinely understood what is being asked of them might matter a great deal in this judgment. Finally, ethical review committees must decide whether to assess study designs strictly on the basis of their effect on study participants, or should also take into account broader issues, such as the relevance of the research to the existing body of knowledge or to the health needs of the people among whom it will be done.

Suggested readings

Allmark P, Mason S. Should Desperate Volunteers be Included in Randomized Controlled Trials? *Journal of Medical Ethics* 2006;32:548-553.

"Randomised controlled trials (RCTs) sometimes recruit participants who are desperate to receive the experimental treatment. This paper defends the practice against three arguments that suggest it is unethical: first, desperate volunteers are not in equipoise. Second, clinicians entering patients into trials are disavowing their therapeutic obligation to deliver the best treatment; they are following trial protocols rather than delivering individualised care. […] Third, desperate volunteers do not give proper consent: effectively, they are coerced."

http://dx.doi.org/10.1136/jme.2005.014282
(accessed 25 August 2008)

Marshall PA. Ethical Challenges in Study Design and Informed Consent for Health Research in Resource-poor Settings. Geneva, Switzerland: WHO/TDR, 2007.

"This review considers ethical challenges to research design and informed consent in biomedical and behavioural studies conducted in resource-poor settings. A review of the literature explores relevant social, cultural, and ethical issues in the conduct of biomedical and social health research in developing countries. Ten case vignettes illustrate ethical challenges that arise in international research with culturally diverse populations." Recommendations are offered to researchers and policy-makers concerned with ethical practices in multinational studies conducted in resource-poor settings.

https://www.who.int/tdr/publications/tdr-research-publications/ethical-challenges-study-design/pdf/ethical_challenges.pdf (accessed 30 August 2008)

Van den Borne F. Using Mystery Clients to Assess Condom Negotiation in Malawi: Some Ethical Concerns. *Studies in Family Planning* 2007;38[4].

"Although most international ethical research codes prescribe the informed consent of research subjects, the present author, as principal investigator for that study, included the mystery client method, which omits informants' consent. […] This article is intended to contribute to the dialogue and debate on ethical research involving mystery clients and to encourage other researchers to share their ethical dilemmas and show how they have addressed them."

http://dx.doi.org/10.1111/j.1728-4465.2007.00144.x
(accessed 25 August 2008)

Weiger C, et al. For and against: Clinical Equipoise and Not the Uncertainty Principle is the Moral Underpinning of the Randomised Controlled Trial. *British Medical Journal*, 2000; 321:756-758.

"The ethical basis for entering patients in randomised controlled trials is under debate. Some doctors espouse the uncertainty principle whereby randomisation to treatment is acceptable when an individual doctor is genuinely unsure which treatment is best for a patient. Others believe that clinical equipoise, reflecting collective professional uncertainty over treatment, is the soundest ethical criterion." While uncertainty is a basic ethical requirement principle for RCTs, this article debates what is meant by uncertainty in a research context.

http://dx.doi.org/10.1136/bmj.321.7263.756
(accessed 25 August 2008)

Case 5

Referral of severely ill children to hospital

Globally, nearly 10 million children younger than 5 years die each year with the vast majority of these deaths occurring in developing countries. Seventy percent are due to acute respiratory infections, diarrhoeal diseases, malaria, measles, malnutrition, or some combination of these. The Integrated Management of Childhood Illness (IMCI) strategy was developed by WHO and the United Nations Children's Fund (UNICEF) in 1992, with the aim of reducing the mortality and morbidity associated with the major causes of childhood illness. IMCI seeks to do this by developing sets of generic guidelines for the management of childhood illnesses at all levels of care, from home to clinic to hospital. Each country can then adapt the guidelines to its own specific situation.

A study is being conducted in South-East Asia to look at the numbers and outcomes of severely ill children who have been referred to a hospital by first-level facility (village clinics/health posts). The objectives of the study are to determine:

- the percentage of children younger than 5 years seen at first-level facilities who are urgently referred to hospital by health workers using the IMCI guidelines;

- the percentage of children referred by health workers who successfully access a referral hospital;

- the percentage of those children judged by a hospital physician to require admission;

- to identify important factors constraining access to referral care for the children judged by first-level health workers as needing an urgent referral to hospital.

Researchers opt for a prospective study design to monitor the referred children's access to hospital care and to identify factors that facilitate or constrain access. In addition to collecting quantitative data on referrals and admissions from first level facility records, the researchers plan to interview the caregivers of the children who are referred to hospital. They believe this will provide them with important additional information about hospital access and outcomes.

The researchers recognize that delaying these interviews until later in the progression of children's illnesses may result in a recall bias on the caregivers' part about access to hospital care. A brief initial interview will, therefore, be conducted in the first-level facility to ask caregivers about their understanding or experience of accessing hospital care. However, to avoid interfering with access for those needing urgent care, the researchers plan follow-up home visits to interview the children's caregivers in more depth. These interviews are to be conducted on the third day after the referral for children who had not yet accessed a hospital; the caregivers of these children will be offered assistance in getting to a hospital. For those children who had accessed a hospital within two days of the referral, home visits and caregiver interviews will be conducted within two weeks of the initial health-facility visit.

Questions

1. Does this study pose an ethical dilemma?

2. Does the presence of study personnel and their interaction with children's caregivers at the first-level facilities oblige them to offer help that wouldn't otherwise be available?

3. What type of assistance, if any, should be offered to children's caregivers? Should the caregivers be given monetary or other assistance that would help the children to gain access to the hospitals if this assistance will not be sustained once the study is finished?

Adapted from: "Referral of Severely Ill Children to Hospital", contributed by Nancy Kass and Joan Atkinson, Johns Hopkins Bloomberg School of Public Health and Johns Hopkins Berman Institute of Bioethics.

Case 6

Negotiating safe sex practices

Dr J, a European anthropologist who has extensive experience in a west African country, designed a study in that country to examine whether and how women involved in the sex trade negotiate condom use by their male partners. Information about this behaviour might help to reduce the incidence of HIV/AIDS in this population. The study investigated the sex trade in and around places of urban entertainment (i.e. bars, bottle stores, and discos). Dr J was concerned that if women were asked directly they might not provide truthful answers about their condom practices. Therefore, the study used a form of participant-observation that depended on deception. Research associates doubled up as fake male "customers", and were trained, supervised, and debriefed daily. They casually met women in one of the venues, presumably to "negotiate for sex", and asked them how, why, and with whom these women bartered casual sex. Before their "deal" was completed, a confederate fake client intervened, which offered the research associate an excuse not to have sex.

Dr J submitted her research proposal to the research ethics committee of the country's health ministry for prior review and approval. The board members concluded that the research would produce reliable information on the views of these women about HIV/AIDS, their sexual practices, and their condom negotiation skills, and that this information would provide a basis for better policy-making. Some members of the committee, however, were concerned that the fake clients would "waste" the women's time, causing them financial losses. The research ethics committee therefore decided to approve the study on the condition that the fake customers would compensate the women for their "lost opportunities" by leaving them money.

However, when an article describing the field methodology, findings, and ethical implications is submitted to an international journal, the reviewers and editor judge that the research method breaches the ethical code – the fake customers had misled research participants, notwithstanding the approval of the research ethics committee. When informed of this, the committee members reiterate their support for the research; they feel justified in disregarding the "Western" code.

Questions

1. Was Dr J justified in using her research design? Whether or not you find this research design justifiable, could another study design have produced findings that were as good or better?

2. Using the same study design, what additional advice could the research ethics committee have given to the investigator to improve the conduct of the study?

3. If the health ministry's research ethics committee found the study ethically justified and useful and hence approved it, should the journal have accepted the article for publication rather than apply an ethical code which the researchers and the REC don't agree with?

4. International ethics guidelines recommend that research participants should be informed about the findings of the research once a study is over and that this should occur in a manner which will allow them to understand the research outcomes and possibly benefit from them. What issues might arise in this case when the study results are conveyed to the research participants?

Based on: van der Geest S. Confidentiality and Pseudonyms: A Fieldwork Dilemma from Ghana. Anthropology Today 2003, 19:14-18.

Case 7

Investigating treatment recommendations

An investigator at an infectious-disease hospital in a south Asian country wants to know what remedies drug sellers and pharmacists are recommending for the treatment of diarrhoea, in order to develop educational materials for both the drug sellers and patients.

The investigator believes that drug sellers would not answer him truthfully if he identifies himself as a researcher before interviewing them, and so decides to undertake a study that requires some deception. He proposes to employ four young men, dressed as villagers, to individually approach a number of different drug sellers for advice on how to treat a 2-year old boy who is at home with fever and green, watery diarrhoea. These men would then purchase the drugs recommended by the drug seller. He plans that the four men would continue their survey for a week, visiting up to six shops each. The shops would not be identified in the subsequent report. None of the drug sellers would know the actual purpose or identity of the buyers; nor would they be aware of their own status as anonymous, non-consenting participants in a research study.

After the week of purchasing, the products would be catalogued and a report written. If any drug seller had recommended drugs that could place customers at risk, the investigator would undertake an educational intervention with that drug seller.

Questions

1. Do the drug sellers have a right to know that they are participants in a research study? Would this right be violated by the study, and would the study be unethical in view of this violation?

2. Is it ethical for the investigator to intervene with any drug seller whose recommendations place customers at any risk? What about if the recommendations place customers at great risk? Is the investigator ethically obliged to intervene because of the special knowledge he might obtain through the study?

3. What are the risks to the drug sellers? What are the potential benefits for the community? Does the prospect of these benefits justify these risks?

4. Should the investigator return to debrief all the drug sellers (i.e. describe the research study and explain the rationale for their action) after the week-long shopping survey is completed?

Case 8

Testing a new HBV vaccine

Of the five hepatitis viruses, hepatitis B (HBV) is the most serious since it can cause lifelong infections that place victims at high risk of death from cirrhosis of the liver and liver cancer – diseases that kill about a million people every year. Chronic HBV infections are most common in developing countries where most people who have the virus are infected during childhood through perinatal mother-to-child transmission or child-to-child transmission. Vaccines have been exceptionally effective for preventing chronic infections from developing but the cost has deterred their general distribution to children in high incidence, low-income countries.

Two general types of hepatitis B vaccine have been widely used: plasma-derived vaccine and recombinant vaccine. The source of immunogens (HBsAg) used in these vaccines is different. The plasma-derived vaccine obtains HBsAg from the serum of persons chronically infected with HBV. The recombinant vaccine is produced using recombinant DNA technology and the HBsAg obtained is highly purified and inactivated.

Plasma-derived hepatitis B vaccine has been shown to be highly immunogenic and effective for prevention of acute and chronic HBV infection in infants, children, and adults. However, since the first reported case of HIV infection in 1981, safety concerns about plasma-derived vaccines have increased. New-generation recombinant vaccines have, however, proven as effective as plasma-derived vaccines in preventing HBV infection while avoiding potential transmission of HIV and other unknown agents associated with plasma-derived vaccines.

A North American company has developed a novel hepatitis B recombinant vaccine. Phase I and II trials have demonstrated that the vaccine is safe, and preliminary results of a Phase III clinical trial have indicated good immune efficacy and safety in children and adults. Asia is a hyperendemic area for HBV infection, and the government of a large Asian country has approved an application to conduct a clinical trial of the vaccine in its jurisdiction. An institute in one of its largest cities has been provided with the resources to carry out a randomized, double-blind study with one experimental group and two control groups. The experimental group would receive the recombinant HBV vaccine, one control group would receive the plasma-derived HBV vaccine, and the second control group would receive a placebo.

Four hospitals in the city enrolled 240 infants born to HBsAg positive mothers, and therefore at high risk of becoming infected. The researchers briefed the infants' parents about the study, and explained the purpose and procedure of the research. For each child, at least one parent had to provide permission before their child could enrol in the study. The infants received the vaccine at birth, and then at 1 and 6 months of age. At 7 months after birth, a follow-up of each subject to evaluate the safety and protective efficacy of the vaccines took place. At the time the study was carried out, immunization with HBV vaccine was a paid service and was not covered by the national Expanded Programme on Immunization. The coverage rate of HBV vaccination was less than 20% in the city, which was located in the most highly developed area of the country.

Questions

1. Is it ethical to set up the placebo control since 80% of the local children would not otherwise have received a HBV vaccine outside of this trial?

2. If you do not think the study meets current ethical standards, how could it be improved to conform to these standards?

3. Is it sufficient for investigators to seek permission from one parent of each child or should both parents have to agree before a child could be entered in the vaccine trial?

Case 9

Tuberculosis prevention in HIV-positive people

> Although this case is based on research that happened more than a decade ago, it is included here because similar ethical questions arise in contemporary clinical trials.

Pulmonary Tuberculosis (TB) is a highly contagious lung disease which, like the common cold, is spread by the transfer of germs from an infected person to a non-infected person. Many people infected with the TB germ, known as tubercle bacilli, have immune systems which "wall off" the bacilli, and allow the disease to lie dormant for years. Any weakening of the immune system will increase the likelihood of becoming sick with TB. About 5-10% of those who are infected with the germ will develop active TB at some point in life; for people who are HIV-positive the chances are much higher. TB is, in fact, a leading cause of death among people who are HIV-positive.

Isoniazid (INH), rifampin, and pyrazinamide are safe and effective anti-tuberculosis medications used routinely worldwide for treating active TB disease. For HIV negative persons with latent (inactive) TB infection, INH is the recommended standard of care for preventing TB disease in those at high risk of contracting the disease. Use of INH to prevent TB varies from country to country depending upon financial constraints, policy, ability to identify high-risk individuals, and capacity of the health care system. In 1994, the American Thoracic Society and Centres for Disease Control and Prevention stated that in the United States of America, in HIV infected persons with latent TB infection, preventive therapy with isoniazid should be given. This was not the national policy of any developing country at the time.

The usual duration of INH prophylactic therapy is 6-12 months, and thus, many have discussed a shorter regimen to improve adherence to the preventive therapy. From 1993 to 1995, researchers from a North American university collaborated with researchers in Africa to evaluate the safety and efficacy of two shorter (but more expensive) regimens to prevent TB in HIV-infected adults. They also addressed whether TB preventive therapy was even effective in settings where the risk of becoming re-infected with TB was high. A randomized, placebo-controlled clinical trial was conducted among 3000 African HIV-positive adults who were free of TB but determined to be at high risk for developing the disease. Participants were randomly assigned to one of four regimens: placebo (control group); INH daily for 6 months (standard therapy group); INH and rifampin daily for 3 months (test group 1); or INH, rifampin, and pyrazinamide daily for 3 months (test group 2). A placebo design was selected based on the rationale that though INH is known to be safe and effective in preventing TB in HIV negative persons and is routinely administered in many settings, the authors postulated that it may not be safe in HIV-positive persons "because of the enhanced drug hypersensitivity associated with HIV infection", and may not be effective because of re-infection. Participants received monthly supplies of study medications to be self-administered. All participants gave oral informed consent before screening and enrolment in the trial. The study was designed to follow participants for at least 3 years.

Questions

1. Was the use of a placebo justified in this study? Explain.

2. How does the use of placebo in a setting where "no treatment" is the standard of care differ ethically from simply providing no treatment?

3. Given that the multi-drug regimen, even if found to be equally effective, is expected to be much more expensive than the INH alone regimen, and hence unlikely to be affordable or accessible to most in need, should this study have been conducted in Africa? Could this study have been carried out in countries where the cost of the treatment might not have been an issue?

Adapted from: "Placebo and TB", a case study contributed by Joan Atkinson and Nancy Kass, Johns Hopkins Bloomberg School of Public Health and Johns Hopkins Berman Institute of Bioethics.

Case 10

Developing a vaccine for malaria

In the past decade, the rapid rise in the incidence of malaria has been so alarming that it is considered a re-emerging disease. In 2006 alone, an estimated 250-300 million cases resulted in almost a million deaths worldwide. Many of those who die are children: malaria kills one child every 30 seconds. Countries in tropical Africa account for more than 90% of the total malaria incidence and for the great majority of malaria deaths. Factors that contribute to the worsening global malaria situation include the spread of drug-resistant strains, frequent civil unrest in Africa forcing resettlement in endemic areas, gross inadequacy of funds for implementing vector control programmes and providing basic health care, and changing rainfall patterns.

Since malaria is concentrated in the world's poorest countries, which lack well-developed and accessible health care infrastructures, most people needing rapid diagnosis and treatment for malaria don't get it even though the cost per patient may be extremely low by the standards of high-income countries. Historically, vaccines are one of the most cost-effective and sustainable ways to control infectious diseases. Consequently, much malaria research is focused on developing an effective vaccine. Current efforts are concentrating on DNA technologies that might induce an immune response to the different stages of malaria infection. To be effective, any intervention, whether preventive or curative, must be inexpensive and relatively easy to administer and maintain.

A North American university is in the process of designing trials to test a multi-stage DNA vaccine. Preliminary studies in the United States of America have been encouraging; immunization of human research participants shows evidence of a strong immune response, and experimental challenge studies in North American volunteers are being initiated. Larger-scale field studies, for Phases II and III, are being planned due to the acute need to find an effective vaccine as soon as possible. If the vaccine were found to be efficacious in malaria-endemic areas, it could potentially save millions of lives.

A country in sub-Saharan Africa where malaria is endemic has expressed interest in participating in the vaccine research effort. The African and North American investigators begin to work together to design a study protocol to assess the vaccine's efficacy for reducing deaths due to malaria in children younger than 5 years, and particularly in infants. It is thought that the vaccine might work in two possible ways: first, it might prevent vaccinated individuals from getting malaria at all. Second, it might not prevent the acquisition of malaria, but it might prevent those who become infected from becoming seriously ill and/or dying; that is, vaccinated children might get a milder case of malaria.

One of the districts in the country, whose total population is approximately 150 000, has put together a very effective epidemiological surveillance system. Trained community health workers visit each home in every village in the district every three months and record all births, deaths, major illnesses, marriages, and migrations. A centralized, computerized, record keeping system is regularly updated on the basis of the community health worker reports. At the same time, most of the villages in this district are remote and only four health posts serve the entire population. Furthermore, in addition to the high malaria burden (18% of annual income lost due to the disease), trained health care workers, lab facilities, and medicines are in extremely short supply. Children younger than 5 years in the study area suffer an average of six bouts of malaria a year; and fatally afflicted children and infants often die less than 72 hours after developing symptoms

The investigators plan on randomly selecting potential participants (children less than 5 years old) for the vaccine trial from the database gathered by the community health workers. A study vaccination team will visit each home, explain the study, and obtain informed consent from the appropriate caregiver and administer the vaccine or placebo, in double-blind fashion, to those children whose parents agree to participate.

The risks of vaccination are minor, and the potential benefit is prevention of morbidity or mortality due to malaria. The team will then leave the village without implementing any other interventions. The data on subsequent illness and death due to malaria will be collected passively by using the information from the centralized data base that is already in place, as well as active surveillance regularly conducted by the community health workers. The impact on the existing health care structure will be minimal.

Since there is no clearly defined immunological marker to measure protective immunity against malaria, and since mortality is by far the most important outcome variable to measure, the study will look at deaths (and, to the extent that health records and verbal autopsies allow, deaths due to malaria) as a study endpoint. Practically, this means that in the absence of a surrogate marker for mortality, the investigators cannot interfere with the "natural" consequences of malaria transmission in the study villages. Yet, the study investigators are aware that due to the presence of the study itself and with relatively little expense, all or nearly all deaths from malaria in the study population could be avoided. If they identified and treated all cases of malaria in the study population, however, they cannot measure the efficacy of the vaccine, which, of course, is the entire reason for the study.

Questions

1. Is the use of a placebo appropriate in this context? Is there a more appropriate design? If you were a member of the research ethics committee, would you approve this study? Why or why not? On what did you base your decision?

2. Should the investigators provide treatment for malaria cases in the community? If yes, would treatment need to be provided to the entire village taking part in the study? Or only to the infants who develop malaria?

3. Do the investigators have any other duty of care to the research participants or their family members?

4. Is death the only important measure of vaccine success? Given that the diagnosis of malaria is presumptive in most cases and verbal autopsy is used to attribute cause of death, is the trial to substantiate vaccine efficacy justified?

5. Sometimes ethical considerations can affect study design. In this study, how does the ethical obligation of improving malaria care and treatment affect the study design?

6. The case study does not indicate that any provision has been made for an ethical review by the country where the research is being conducted. If the North American partners insist that the review conducted in the United States of America is adequate, what should the host country do? In the host country, who has the ethical obligation to ensure review by a local committee – researchers, government health staff, public health authorities, regulatory bodies, or others? If the host country does not have the capacity to provide ethical oversight, what options are available?

Adapted from: "Malaria Vaccine", a case study contributed by Nancy Kass and Liza Dawson, Johns Hopkins Bloomberg School of Public Health and Johns Hopkins Berman Institute of Bioethics.

Case 11

Should race be listed as a risk factor?

Records from the sexually transmitted infection (STI) clinic at the largest general hospital in a southern African country indicate that the segment of the population self-ascribed as "coloured" has twice as many cases of STIs as the segment that is self-ascribed as "black". By contrast, for almost all other conditions seen in the hospital's outpatient department, the number of cases of a disease in each racial and ethnic group is proportional to that group's percentage of the general population. Even after controlling for socioeconomic status, this distinction in the distribution of STIs remains.

Before the country's independence, government officials assigned individuals to one of four racial categories – black, white, coloured, and Asian – on the basis of factors such as physical appearance, descent, language, and behaviour. Since independence, an individual's membership to one of these racial groups, or a new alternative, "other," is self-ascribed. Authorities may investigate an individual's self-categorization if they suspect them of self-identifying to a racial group to accrue some particular benefit.

Dr Chingana, director of the STI clinic, believes that the disproportionate rate of cases in people who have identified themselves as "coloured", compared with those who have identified as being "black", reflects differences in each group's biological susceptibility to these diseases: he is, however, unsure of the underlying mechanism responsible. Seeking to bolster the evidence supporting this hypothesis, Dr Chingana develops a survey designed to link STI symptoms with a variety of risk factors, including race[1] and ethnicity[2]. He presents his protocol to his institution's research ethics committee for approval.

Ms Johnson, a community representative on the committee who self-identifies as coloured, objects to the inclusion of race as a targeted factor in the survey. She argues that the coloured population is already stigmatized by stereotypes that portray them as promiscuous and lax in using health services. She contends that a finding of higher rates of STI cases in the coloured population will only serve to reinforce these deeply held prejudices. Further, she is sceptical of the notion that being coloured might increase one's risk of contracting an STI and probes for further explanation. Do the bacteria behave differently in coloured people? Is their anatomy different? She wants the race and ethnicity question removed from the questionnaire.

Dr Chingana argues that this question is critical to the study. Moreover, the findings might point to further research that could aid in the development of programmes for STI control aimed at reducing the high rate of infection among coloured people.

Questions

1. Do you agree with Dr Chingana or Ms Johnson? Is it the researchers' responsibility to put safeguards in place to discourage possible stigma?

2. Given that the racial categories were originally, and continue to be, political constructs, should they be used in a scientific study such as this?

3. Given that a hypothesis must be based on more than a vague notion, was the information from the clinic records enough? How could Dr Chingana have strengthened his research protocol?

---

[1] As used here, "race" refers to a group of people connected by common descent or origin.

[2] "Ethnicity" here refers to the culture and/or collective identity shared by a group of people of common descent or origin.

Case 12

Short-course AZT to prevent mother-to-child transmission of HIV

The risk of vertical transmission of HIV during pregnancy and delivery has been estimated at 15-30%, depending on several factors, including the stage of the mother's illness and whether it has been treated. In the mid-1990s, the best-known method for prevention of maternal HIV transmission was the "076 regimen", or long-course AZT treatment, in which a pregnant HIV-positive woman received zidovudine (AZT) five times a day orally from weeks 14 to 34 of the pregnancy and intravenously at the time of delivery. The infant would also be given AZT orally four times a day for 6 weeks after delivery. This regimen reduces vertical transmission of HIV by about 68%, provided that breastfeeding does not occur.[1]

However most public health experts in sub-Saharan Africa at the time that the study was designed considered that the "076" long-course regimen was impractical, because:

- prenatal visits do not begin until just before delivery;

- most deliveries do not occur in hospital, and of those that do, intravenous infusion during labour is not viable for most; and

- the cost of AZT for the long-course treatment is not affordable for most patients in most countries in sub-Saharan Africa.

To address these barriers, researchers proposed a series of multi-site, placebo-controlled trials in sub-Saharan Africa and the Asia-Pacific region to evaluate the efficacy of a short course of AZT for the prevention of vertical transmission of HIV. Participating mothers would begin treatment with AZT or a placebo 2 days before delivery; infants would also receive the drug (or placebo) for 2 days postpartum. The researchers were uncertain whether the short course would be as effective as the long course; however, a short course of treatment would be much less expensive than a long course and could increase access to care because it would be more in accord with delivery patterns in these two regions. Even if the short-course regimen proved less effective than the long-course regimen, the researchers hoped the short course would be adopted as standard preventive therapy in the absence of other feasible alternative regimens.

The researchers proposed to use a placebo control, since:

- the clinically relevant comparison was with the treatment that pregnant women were receiving at the time, which was no treatment at all;

- due to the practical and financial barriers, the long-course regimen would not be widely implemented, and thus local public health officials in the study countries found it unethical to provide it to the control groups in the clinical trials; and

- because the short-course regimen requires less time to complete, the study countries could adopt the short course much sooner if it proved effective.

Critics, mainly in the West, argued that the control groups should be given the "076" regimen rather than a placebo, because:

- the decision to use a placebo, rather than long-course treatment in the control groups, violated the explicit provisions of the *Declaration of Helsinki*;[2]

---

[1] WHO recommends that HIV-infected women should use exclusive breastfeeding for the first 6 months of a child's life unless replacement feeding is acceptable, feasible, affordable, sustainable, and safe for them and their infants before that time. If those criteria are met, avoidance of all breastfeeding by HIV-infected women is recommended. WHO HIV and Infant Feeding Technical consultation. Consensus Statement. Geneva, Switzerland: Inter-agency Task Team (IATT) on Prevention of HIV Infections in Pregnant Women, Mothers and their Infants, 2006.

[2] In June 1964, the World Medical Association (WMA) adopted the "Declaration of Helsinki: Ethical Principles for Medical Research Involving Human Subjects. Although the original version did not address the issue of placebos, the issue emerged in subsequent revisions. Paragraph 32 in the 2008 version (based upon paragraph 29 in the earlier 2004 version) states that "The benefits, risks, burdens and effectiveness of a new method should be tested against those of the best proven current method, except in the following circumstances:

- The use of placebo, or no treatment, is acceptable in studies where no proven current method exists; or

- Where for compelling and scientifically sound methodological reasons the use of placebo is necessary to determine the efficacy or safety of a method and the patients who receive placebo or no treatment will not be subject to any additional risk of serious or irreversible harm."
For more information, visit http://www.wma.net/e/policy/b3.htm (accessed 5 June 2009).

- the researchers were using a double standard since they would not be permitted to run a placebo-controlled trial in their own countries, on the ground that an effective therapy existed; and

- even though results would take longer – and be more expensive – to achieve with active rather than placebo controls, trials could be designed that excluded placebo controls.

Questions

1. If the health authorities in the African and Asia-Pacific countries declared the proven effectiveness of long-course treatment irrelevant and impractical to their needs, should research ethics committees in the donor institutions still insist on long-course treatment for the controls?

2. If the researchers believed that short-course AZT would be effective but less so than long-course treatment, should the short course have been tested at all (even if the control group received the long course)?

3. If the test could not be conducted in a high-income country, would this, by definition, lead to a double standard for therapeutic intervention?

Adapted from a case study provided to the Harvard University School of Public Health by the Case Program, John F. Kennedy School of Government, Harvard University

Case 13

Testing an ayurvedic medicine for malaria

Malaria is a major health problem in many areas of South Asia. Due largely to problems of drug resistance and treatment failure of chloroquine,[1] a common therapy for *Plasmodium falciparum* and *Plasmodium vivax* malaria,[2] there is great interest in exploring new drugs, drug combinations, and/or indigenous remedies to combat these malarial agents.

Ayush-64 is a combination of four Ayurvedic drugs which are mixed and then formulated into 500 mg tablets.[3] This combination is patented and registered to a national traditional medicine research centre in South Asia. Ayush 64 has not undergone any animal toxicity or preclinical toxicity studies, since its individual components have been used in human beings over many hundred years. The formulation itself has been used for treatment of malaria over several decades by physicians who practise traditional medicine. A study conducted more than 20 years ago reported that Ayush-64 was effective against malaria. In the original study of the formulation, patients who received clinical diagnoses of malaria were allowed to participate, however, the assessment criteria were not uniform and neither cases nor clinical success was confirmed by laboratory tests. Thus, in order to introduce Ayush-64 into the national malaria program, it was necessary to retest the drug.

The centre responsible for malaria research in the capital city oversaw the new Ayush-64 trials. Following approval for the research study from the malaria research centre's research ethics committee, the study commenced at the research centre and various national anti-malaria programme clinics, which had been selected as study sites. Patients from four to five periurban, low socioeconomic villages and resettlement colonies attend these clinics. Those with proven cases of *P. vivax* malaria who sought treatment at the clinics were asked to volunteer for the study if they also met the following criteria: 18-60 years of age, with asexual parasitaemia of less than 50 000 per μl, and febrile or had a history of fever within the past 48 hours. Pregnant and lactating women, those people with glucose-6 phosphate dehydrogenase deficiency, and those who took antimalarials in the 7 days before their clinic visit were excluded from the study. Patients who met these inclusion criteria were enrolled after providing written informed consent.

Patients were randomly allocated to one of two treatment regimens. One group received a total dose of 1500 mg of chloroquine given over 3 days, followed by 15 mg primaquine[4] daily for 5 days. This is the nationally recommended treatment for *P. vivax* malaria in that country. The other group received Ayush-64 in three daily doses of two 500 mg tablets for 5 days. Patient response to the Ayush-64 was determined by the presence or absence of parasites in the peripheral smear on day 5. Non-responsive patients received the same medications for another 2 days, after which, if they remained positive they were labelled as treatment failures, and given the control treatment (chloroquine followed by primaquine). The dosage of Ayush-64 was in accordance with the doses used in the earlier study. All patients who became positive after having a negative smear at day 7 were labelled as recrudescences. Patients were followed as outpatients for 28 days for clinical and parasitological cure. No attempt was made to follow up patients who dropped out of the study.

---

[1] A drug long used for treatment and prevention of malaria. Over time, the malaria parasite *Plasmodium falciparum* has developed widespread resistance against chloroquine.

[2] There are four types of human malaria – Plasmodium falciparum, P. vivax, P. malariae, and P. ovale, The most deadly type of malaria infection is P. falciparum, which together with P. vivax, is also the most common.

[3] Ayurveda and Siddha are two forms of traditional medicine recognized and licensed in India. Ayurveda is based on the use of herbal preparations, and Siddha is based on the use of the preparations of various metals. The word "Ayurveda" is a derived from the sanskrit words āyus meaning "life," "life principle," or "long life" and the word veda, which refers to a system of "knowledge." Ayurveda means 'the knowledge needed for long life'. According to the Ayurveda principles, health or sickness depends on the presence or absence of a balanced state of the total body matrix including the balance between its different constituents. Both the intrinsic and extrinsic factors can cause disturbance in the natural equilibrium giving rise to disease. This loss of equilibrium can happen by dietary indiscrimination, undesirable habits and non-observance of rules of healthy living. The treatment consists of restoring the balance of disturbed body-mind matrix through regulating diet, correcting life-routine and behaviour, administration of drugs and resorting to preventive therapy.
From http://indianmedicine.nic.in/ayurveda.asp (accessed on 9 May 2008).

[4] A drug used to treat the *Plasmodium vivax* or *ovale* variants of malaria. Primaquine only attacks malarial parasites in tissue and therefore is usually administered in combination with treatments that target parasites in the bloodstream. If primaquine is not administered there is a very high likelihood of a *P. vivax* relapse within weeks or months, sometimes even years.

Questions

1. What evidence is necessary for a treatment to be tested in human participants? Was there enough evidence in this case to test Ayush-64? Should this evidence be different if the treatment in question is labelled a traditional therapy?

2. Was it ethical to conduct the study? Why or why not? What are the ethical issues raised by the study design?

3. What was the responsibility of the researchers to patients who dropped out of the study?

Case 14

Evaluating the use of traditional medicines for diarrhoea

Hydrocotyle asiatica, or 'thankuni', is a plant common to South Asia which, when dried, ground up, and added to water, is reported to be effective for treatment of bloody diarrhoea. 'Thankuni' is the main ingredient of a popular traditional medicine, 'ajorno', which is produced by a local company. This medicine is widely available, very popular, and quite inexpensive. A paper suggesting that 'thankuni' decreases bloody diarrhoea appeared in an unrefereed journal from an institute of traditional medicine in South Asia. However, no clinical studies have been conducted on this product, and the specific chemical composition has not been determined

Dr Wabano, an investigator at an international research institution, is intrigued by this product, and wants to evaluate its clinical effectiveness. The present treatments for dysentery[1] (by far the most common cause of bloody diarrhoea in South Asia) are fluid intake and norfloxacin,[2] an antibiotic that is clinically effective and bactericidal. Norfloxacin, however, is often unavailable outside the major cities (80% of the population is rural) and, even when it is available, is too expensive for many people to afford. Dr Wabano reasons that if the traditional medicine proves effective, therapy will be more accessible to everyone because of availability and cost.

The investigator submits a protocol to the study committee of the institute for a double-blinded study that compares the clinical effectiveness and bactericidal properties of 'ajorno' with norfloxacin. Adult patients admitted or seen on an outpatient basis with a history of dysentery will be randomly assigned to one of the treatment groups after a rectal swab has been taken for a bacteriological diagnosis. 'Ajorno', which is in a powdered form, will be put into a gelatine capsule so that it is indistinguishable from the antibiotic.

The ethics review committee meets, and votes not to approve the protocol for the following reasons:

- The specific chemical composition of 'ajorno' (i.e. "thankuni") is not known.

- The prior reports of effectiveness have been for "bloody diarrhoea" which might include any number of diagnoses, including dysentery and amoebiasis.

- No studies in peer-reviewed journals report that the traditional medicine is effective or suggest a mechanism for its reputed effectiveness.

Dr Wabano notes that it would be next to impossible to define all of the ingredients of this traditional medicine, and that if attempted, this would be a costly undertaking. He suggests that those on the review panel who voted against approval were biased against traditional medicines, and have denigrated the indigenous science of the country, and tried to impose their own "western biases" on scientific research.

Questions

1. In your opinion, was the research ethics committee correct in its assessment? Why or why not? Is there an alternative study design that the committee could recommend?

2. Is the investigator correct in his accusation that members of the committee who voted against the approval of the study are showing a "western bias" in their decision?

3. If the study were approved as presented above, would the committee have used a double standard in its assessment of the ethics of the design?

4. In circumstances where the researcher and the research ethics committee disagree, how might the situation be mediated?

---

[1] Any of various disorders marked by inflammation of the intestines, especially of the colon, and attended by abdominal pain, and frequent stools containing blood and mucus. Causes include chemical irritants, bacteria, protozoa and parasitic worms.

[2] An antibiotic used to treat a range of bacterial infections.

Case 15

Twin registry genetics

The extent to which common mental disorders, including alcohol dependency and suicidal ideation, are caused by genetic factors versus environmental ones remains unclear. Promising twin-study research on mental disorders has been conducted in developed countries, but such studies might not be relevant for developing countries.

Collaborating investigators from Europe and South-East Asia design a population twin study to be conducted in a South-East Asian country which has documented high rates of suicide, alcohol dependency, and somatoform disorders[1]. The study sample will include about 2000 twin pairs and 1000 singletons, all between the ages of 18 and 65 years. The only exclusion criteria are severe mental illness and illiteracy. While the primary study goal is to determine causality (nature or nurture) of common mental disorders, a related secondary goal is to document their prevalence.

All participants will be interviewed by trained researchers who will both assess them for common mental disorders (including anxiety, depression, substance dependency, and suicidal ideation) and administer a questionnaire about significant life events, deprivation, poor academic achievement, and early experiences of abuse and/or neglect. The only biological materials that will be taken from the research participants are buccal swabs from same sex twins in order to determine their twin status (monozygosity or dizygosity). After the results of the swab are conveyed to the participants, the DNA samples will be anonymized, coded, and stored. Appropriate informed consent will be obtained from participants for the interviews and for taking the swabs. No reimbursement will be given to the participants for their time and no follow-up will be provided after the initial interview and assessment. During the assessment, those diagnosed with a mental disorder that warrants treatment will be referred to the nearest health facility providing care to people with mental illnesses. In accordance with contemporary national practices, if an individual is found to be at serious risk of suicide or to have severe psychosis with no insight and diminished capacity to consent to treatment, their nearest relative will be contacted to safeguard their health and safety.

Questions

1. Is it acceptable to design a study with exclusion criteria that leave out the illiterate and the severely ill, groups who could be most in need?

2. As some of the research subjects might have mental illnesses detected for the first time during the interview, is it sufficient for the researchers to refer patients to a service without assurance that they will be properly treated and without promise of future follow-up? What are their obligations?

3. Are the researchers responsible for following up on the potential impact that the results of this study might have on individuals who have identical twins with severe mental illnesses?

---

[1] The somatoform disorders are a group of mental disturbances placed in a common category on the basis of their external symptoms. These disorders are characterized by physical complaints that appear to be medical in origin but that cannot be explained in terms of a physical disease, the results of substance abuse, or by another mental disorder.

Case 16

Observing newborn care practices

Each year, about four million infants in developing countries die during their first month of life. Many of these deaths could be prevented by improving newborn care practices such as proper breastfeeding, hygiene, warmth, and quick access to health care.

A group of university researchers in an East Asian country are conducting an observational study that will assist them to develop means to promote more appropriate newborn care; the study is being carried out in a nearby community with a particularly high neonatal mortality rate. After obtaining approval from the university's research ethics committee, the investigators hire field workers to observe current practices in all households that have babies younger than 3 months. This entails observing each baby's environment (cleanliness, warmth), care (clothing, bathing), and interactions with caregivers. The field workers are told to abstain from intervening, and simply to record what they observe.

Informed consent for the observations is obtained from each baby's mother and one other caregiver (either the mother-in-law or the husband). The consent form states that they will neither be compensated for their participation, nor benefit directly from the study, although their community might benefit if the results of the research lead to improvements in practices for care of newborn babies.

As a field worker is recording her observations of a household, she notices that the members of the household are also observing her, apparently looking to her for approval of what they are doing and how they are interacting with the infant. She tries to remain expressionless as she observes the various practices, though she finds this especially difficult as the mother prepares formula for an infant using stored water from the nearby river. She is concerned that the water has not been boiled and that the feed is much too diluted.

Questions

1 Is it ethically appropriate for the field worker simply to observe a practice that she knows could be harmful for the child? If not, when should she interfere?

2 Could this study have been designed differently so as not to put the field worker in a dilemma, while still getting the desired evidence?

3 Generally, what are investigators' obligations to participants in observational studies?

4 Need informed consent be obtained from other people who enter the household during the observation period if they could be observed as they interact with the baby?

Case 17

Compassionate intervention during an observational study

A field worker is conducting observations in households with infants younger than 3 months in an East Asian community with high infant mortality. This is being done as part of an observational study to gather data to generate evidence to promote more appropriate newborn care. The study has been approved by an appropriate research ethics committee. The field workers have been told to abstain from intervening and simply to record what they observe. When they gave their consent to the observation, the baby's mother and a second caregiver were informed that they would not benefit directly from the study, although their community might benefit if the research results lead to improvements in practices for care of newborn babies.

Although she knows she should not intervene, the field worker feels very compassionate towards the families whom she observes and always answers any health-related questions that they pose to the best of her ability. In one household, the field worker is asked for help to treat an older sibling who has been suffering from a high-grade fever for 2 days and is obviously quite sick. The family tells her that they have been unable to gather the resources necessary to take the child to the nearest health facility, which is about 20 km away and is poorly staffed.

The health worker fears that the child will die if the child does not receive immediate care. The field worker is also worried that she will lose support from the villagers if she does not intervene. On the other hand, she is concerned that her help at this stage in the study will result in her being flooded with additional requests for health care assistance.

Questions

1. Should the provision of care that is ancillary to a study's design ever be considered ethically obligatory, and if so, when and why? What reasoning supports your response?

2. How should investigators conducting an observational study deal with the inadequacy of the health care facilities available to research participants and their families? Are the duties relating to interventional studies any different than for observational studies?

3. If the design of a study does not make provision for care of people such as the sibling in this case, would an individual researcher (here, a field worker) have any individual ethical duty to respond affirmatively to a request for care? Does this obligation take precedence over her obligations to the study? In the case of conflicting moral imperatives, what should the field worker do?

4. How might the field worker deal with the dilemma in which she finds herself, when responding compassionately to this family's needs could open her to a flood of further requests, which she would be unable to meet, especially when that might itself affect her ability to continue making observations in the community?

Chapter III

Harm and Benefit

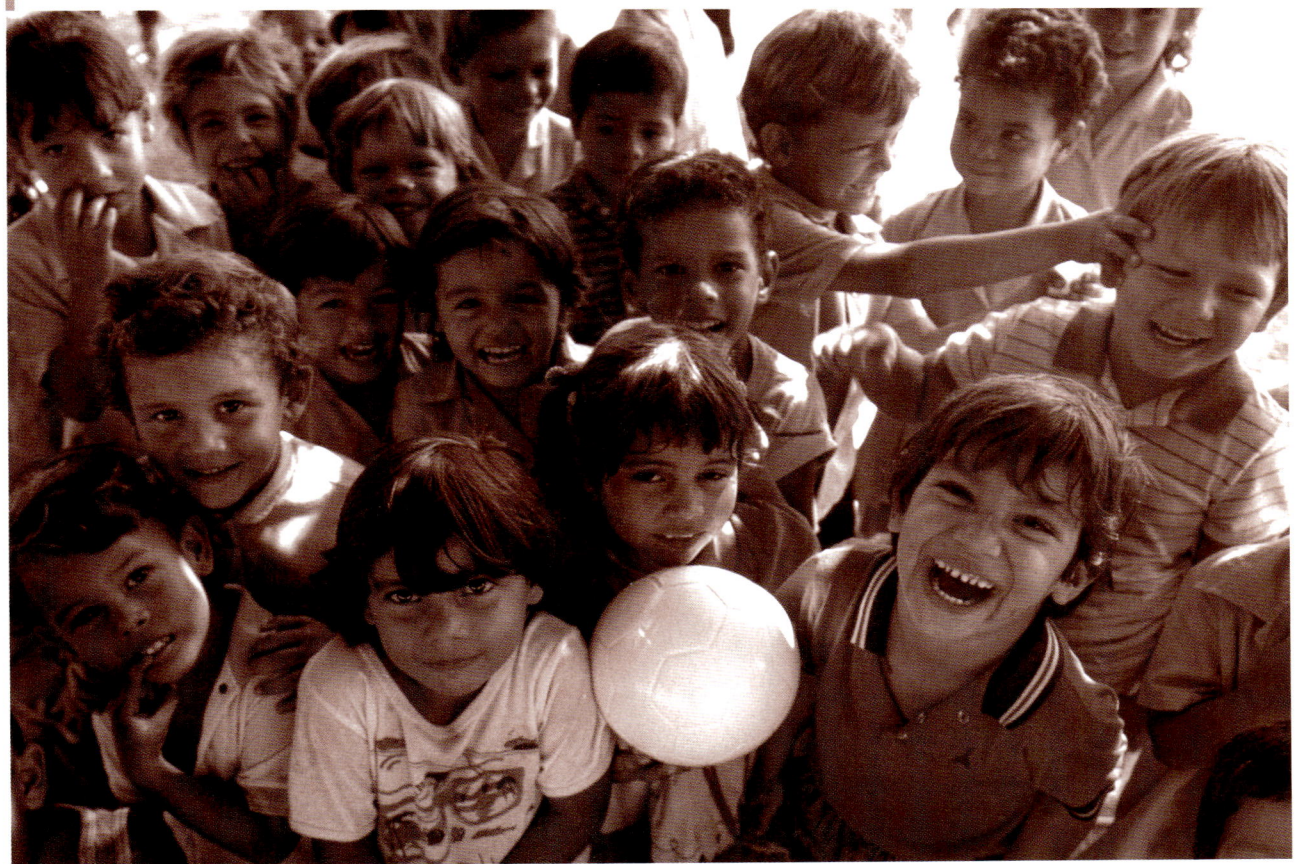

Introduction: Chapter III

Are research benefits and harms fairly distributed?

Research with human participants raises ethical concerns precisely because the research that scientists might need to do in order to obtain useful knowledge might not always serve participants' best interests. When scientific needs coincide with participants' interests, studies are usually unproblematic. In this ideal scenario, people who enrol in research gain otherwise unobtainable advantages and suffer no harms, and the knowledge gained in the process helps to improve health care in the future and adds to the storehouse of scientific knowledge.

Benefits: fairness and justice issues

Ethical questions, however, arise even in these ideal circumstances. For example, if a study involves a potential benefit for participants but little risk of harm, the number of people who wish to participate might be more than the study can accommodate. This raises questions of justice: who should be chosen for participation, and what factors should be used as justification for choosing among individuals or groups? A promising drug, or even slightly better access to health care, are both very good reasons to seek participation in a research study, and investigators should have defensible grounds for the choices they make among prospective enrolees. For example, is there an ethical justification for excluding women of childbearing age or people who are HIV-positive from the possible benefits of the trial? Along the same lines, why would one community be chosen as a research site and not another? These are questions that RECs need to consider during the review of research protocols.

Other benefit-related questions include: who will benefit from the knowledge gained? Why should the limited resources available for research be used to learn about one disease rather than another, or about the health problems of one group instead of another? Is it ethical for sponsors to reap large benefits in the form of patents and profits from drugs that are proven to be effective through research trials, even if the knowledge gained does eventually provide benefits to the population from which the research participants came?

Justice in the distribution of benefits at the completion of the research study should also be considered (see Chapter VI on *Obligations to Participants and Communities*).

Non-reciprocal harm

In research which involves a possible risk to participants, a study's potential harms are generally required to be less than its expected benefits, which include the benefits of the new knowledge to science and to society. The most challenging moral dilemmas about risk and benefit occur when participants are placed at risk of harm, or are burdened by discomfort or distress, without the prospect of any personal benefit. In such cases, the REC must decide whether the expected burden on participants is justified by the prospective benefits to others that could result from the knowledge gained, and whether participants will be appropriately compensated for the harm they could incur by taking part in the research.

There are no easy answers to the question of how REC members should reach these balancing judgments and since this moral balancing is arguably the central task of RECs, it is surprising that it is rarely addressed in academic literature, guidelines, or textbooks. Indeed, little research has been undertaken to ascertain what thresholds, or balance between harms and benefits, if any, are commonly used. In accounts of research abuses, the offending scientists have often clearly overemphasized science at the cost of participants' well-being, but identification of the correct balance needs further attention.

In many studies, all participants face the possibility of harm, distress, or discomfort. For example, in the early phases of testing new drugs (that is, mostly in phase I and II studies), investigators must probe the maximal dose of the experimental drug that human beings can tolerate. As they near such limits, some participants might be harmed or experience discomfort. However, because these early studies are either carried out on healthy volunteers or are being tested for the first time in patients, participants are not expected to receive any corresponding benefits. Even in later phases of clinical trials, the possibility of adverse reactions and outcomes cannot be ruled out, and positive consequences cannot be assured. RECs must ensure that possible harms are minimized and are outweighed by possible benefits and that potential participants will be given a full and honest account of the harms and benefits that they could experience if they agree to join a study. Conscientiously carried out, the consent process should permit prospective participants to weigh the potential for harm against any prospect for benefit.

Comparison of harms and benefits

Potential harms and benefits might be difficult to compare because of uncertainty, because they could affect different people in different ways, or because the harms and benefits are of different kinds (e.g. pain versus extension of life in a test of chemotherapy for cancer). This complicates decisions for individual participants, but RECs must also judge whether the net prospects for participants will be negative (that is, potential harm or discomfort is greater than the corresponding benefit). This might also occur in studies that do not have therapeutic aims for participants (e.g. studies of new diagnostic tests or research on the biological basis of diseases).

Sometimes investigators find emerging trends for the success (or failure) of the drug they are testing so compelling that they face a dilemma about whether or not to continue with the trial. In the past, some investigators did decide to stop a trial early so the treatment being investigated could be made available to participants in the placebo group and to other patients who might benefit. With the double-blind designs now commonly used, a decision to end a trial early usually rests with an independent data and safety monitoring board (DSMB) which has access to the accumulating results of the trial on an unblinded basis and which is guided by stopping rules set in advance for the trial. A DSMB may end a trial because statistically significant results have been achieved before the number of research participants originally planned has been enrolled. Alternatively, it may call off a trial because the pattern of harm (either to the active or the control group) is both great and clear even though not yet statistically significant, which means that the trial results will remain uncertain. (Depending on the situation, another study may or may not be undertaken to clear up the unresolved questions.)

Balancing harms, benefits, and study design – the role of the RECs

As discussed in Chapter II on *Issues in Study Design*, RECs might have to decide whether to trade off scientific certainty in favour of protecting participants. Sometimes, however, research design questions are decided based on a balance of ethical considerations. For example, should a study be undertaken that involves exposing twenty consenting participants to a substantial chance of physical harm, if the same results could be produced by an alternative design which has a much smaller risk of causing harm to individual participants, but which requires two thousand participants? Likewise, should a new vaccine be studied first in older teenagers who are capable of giving consent, and then in younger teenagers who are capable of providing "assent" but not valid consent, in order to develop greater certainty about its safety before it is tested on the infants for whom it is intended but who are too young to give even assent? How can potential harms (and benefits) of various types and magnitudes to different people simply be summed up arithmetically? Are there times when it is not useful to compare harms and benefits – in which case, judgments about the ethics of a study must rest on other grounds?

Balancing risk and benefit is complicated still further when both potential harms and benefits accrue to people other than those enrolled as participants. For example, one concern regarding xenotransplantation (in which animal organs are transplanted into human beings) is that organs could contain hitherto unknown retroviruses that could spread through the human population, in a similar way to HIV. Should RECs take such potential harms into account, or is their purview limited to study participants? This issue arises only rarely in connection with infectious diseases, but more commonly for groups that could be (or could consider themselves to be) adversely affected by the publication of a study's research results. For example, the results of genetic studies can have implications for close relatives of participants. Similarly, in a study of HIV prevalence in several South Asian villages, some residents feared that because the identity of the towns could not be adequately masked, the study would stigmatize all residents as HIV-positive.

Suggested readings

Bayer A, Tadd W. Unjustified Exclusion of Elderly People from Studies Submitted to Ethics Committees for Approval: Descriptive Study. *British Medical Journal*, **2000; 321: 992-993.**

"Ethics committees are in a strong position to influence research practice and to reduce unethical age discrimination. We encourage them to request justification whenever protocols include inappropriate age restrictions – and if this is not forthcoming, approval might be conditional on age limits being removed. This policy would promote more positive attitudes towards elderly people among researchers as well as safer, more effective treatments and services."

http://dx.doi.org/10.1136/bmj.321.7267.992
(accessed 25 August 2008)

Moodley K. Microbicide Research in Developing Countries: Have We Given the Ethical Concerns Due Consideration? *BioMedCentral Medical Ethics*, **2007; 8:10**

"Ethical concerns relating to safety in microbicide research are a major international concern. However, in the urgency to develop a medically efficacious microbicide, some of these concerns may not have been anticipated. In the risk-benefit assessment of research protocols, both medical and psycho-social risk must be considered." This article examines a number of concerns related to safety risks in international microbicide trials.

http://dx.doi.org/10.1186/1472-6939-8-10
(accessed 25 August 2008)

Schenk K, Williamson J. Ethical Approaches to Gathering Information from Children and Adolescents in International Settings – Guidelines and Approaches. Washington, DC, USA: Population Council, 2005.

"Program managers and researchers often gather information from children and adolescents in order to develop and evaluate appropriate responses to their needs. During information gathering, children and adolescents require protection and respect in accordance with the highest ethical standards." This publication draws attention to the many issues which can arise when conducting research with children as participants. The issue of consent and assent is discussed.

http://www.popline.org/docs/1673/299734.html
(accessed 7 April 2009)

Upshur R, Lavery JV, Tindana PO. Taking Tissue Seriously Means Taking Communities Seriously. *BioMedCentral Medical Ethics*, **2007;8:11.**

"In this paper, [the authors] outline the salient ethical issues raised by tissue exportation, review the current ethical guidelines and norms, review the literature on what is known empirically about perceptions and practices with respect to tissue exportation from the developing to the developed world, set out what needs to be known in terms of a research agenda, and outline what needs to be done immediately in terms of setting best practices." The authors conclude that any solution will necessitate going beyond concern with individual level consent to meaningful engagement with communities.

http://dx.doi.org/10.1186/1472-6939-8-11
(accessed 25 August 2008)

Wilmshurst P. Scientific Imperialism. *British Medical Journal*, 1997;314:840-841.

"Should research be conducted in a country where the people are unlikely to benefit from the findings because most of the population is too poor to buy effective treatment? Are poor people in developing countries being exploited in research for the benefit of patients in the developed world where subject recruitment to a randomised trial would be difficult?" This editorial addresses questions of inequality arising when health research is conducted in developing countries.

http://www.bmj.com/cgi/content/full/314/7084/840
(accessed 9 May 2008)

Case 18

Rotavirus vaccine

Rotavirus is one of the most common causes of severe diarrhoeal disease and dehydration in infants and young children in both developed and developing countries. The virus, which infects almost all children by the time they are aged 2 or 3 years, appears to be as prevalent in high-income as in low-income countries despite wide differences in the functioning of their sanitation and health care systems. The difference in income level is instead manifested in a marked difference in the morbidity and mortality rates associated with the virus. Of the estimated 527 000 rotavirus deaths per year, most are among children aged younger than 2 years; and most – up to 85% – are in low-income countries.

The observation that rates of illness caused by rotavirus are universally high among children in both developed and developing countries indicates that making water supplies clean and following good hygiene practices will not markedly decrease the incidence of rotavirus in developing nations. Therefore, further improvements in water or hygiene are unlikely to have a substantial impact on preventing the disease. For this reason, and because of the heavy worldwide burden of disease caused by rotavirus, immunization by vaccine would be an important public health intervention in both developed and developing countries.

Based on the findings of four randomized controlled efficacy trials in the United States of America and northern Europe, in the late 1990s a North American national drug licensing body licensed the quadrivalent rhesus rotavirus vaccine (RRV-TV) for routine vaccination in its own country.

Following that licensure, about a million children received the vaccine. Within a year, the number of reported cases of intussusception[1] among infants vaccinated with RRV-TV, (estimated at one case per 10 000 children vaccinated), raised concerns. The US department of health began to analyze reports from the system set up to monitor and provide post-licensure surveillance of adverse events after vaccination. In the report of its findings, the department of health stated that the data raised "strong concerns" about the relationship between vaccination with RRV-TV and intussusception. Consequently, the department recommended that administration of RRV-TV to children should be postponed. A few months later, the manufacturer of the vaccine voluntarily withdrew RRV-TV from the North American market, which was interpreted by many in developing countries as a sign that the product was unsafe.

There is a view, however, that in developing countries the burden of morbidity and mortality induced by rotavirus outweighs the risk of serious morbidity from the vaccine. If the vaccine is found to be effective, the benefits of the vaccine outweigh the risks. Therefore, the scientific community is equally responsible for deaths caused by withholding the vaccine as for deaths caused by the vaccine itself, and it is unethical not to continue randomized controlled trials of RRV-TV in developing countries. Indeed, not doing such studies would "perpetuate global inequities in access to health care."

The ministry of health of a developing country compares the risk of a child younger than 2 years dying from rotavirus diarrhoea (1/100) with the risk of a rotavirus vaccine-related death, for example from intussusception (1/10 000 vaccines). The ministry concludes that, if affordable, the vaccine should be given to all children within the first 3 months of life. The ministry directs a well-respected state-run pharmaceutical company, LDC Pharma, to obtain the production techniques and rights from the North American manufacturer for local production and distribution. LDC Pharma assures the ministry of health that it can produce the vaccine at an affordable price.

---

[1] The bowel telescoping into itself, cutting off its own blood supply, and potentially leading to obstruction and, if untreated, death.

The North American company, however, refuses to transfer its production techniques to LDC Pharma, even after LDC Pharma assures the company that it will not sell or distribute the rotavirus vaccine outside the country. The North American company notes that it wants to recoup the almost US$ 150 million that it spent on developing the vaccine, and expresses concern that it could potentially be held liable should any complications be associated with the vaccine. Despite the North American company's refusal, however, LDC Pharma could possibly obtain the vaccine production technique by invoking the concept of compulsory licensing.[1] This clause, however, can only be invoked under specific conditions and only if the authorization meets certain requirements.

Questions

1. Assuming that the vaccine is the cause of at least some of the cases of intussusception, should the vaccine be administered in settings where rotavirus is a significant cause of morbidity and mortality in young children? Is there an ethical difference between exposing a "sick" population of children to a possible complication that can cause death, versus a "healthy" population of children?

2. Is there an ethical difference between exposing a population of children that is at a higher risk of dying from (in this case) rotavirus to a possible fatal complication from a vaccine, versus a population of children that normally does not have any serious morbidity from rotavirus infection?

3. What degree of risk is acceptable in this case and who should make that determination?

4. Is the North American manufacturer under any moral or ethical obligation to allow the developing country to produce the vaccine for local consumption?

5. If the North American manufacturer refuses to either produce an affordable rotavirus vaccine for developing countries or give up its patent rights so that it can be produced at a much lower cost in a developing country, are these countries under any moral or ethical obligation to honour these patent rights? (Consider that the World Trade Organization (WTO) Agreement on Trades Related Aspects of Intellectual Property Rights (TRIPS) will, in certain circumstances, allow WTO member states to issue temporary licenses against the will of the patent holder.)

Adapted from a case contributed by Joan Atkinson, Nancy Kass, and Andrea Ruff – Johns Hopkins Bloomberg School of Public Health & Johns Hopkins Berman Institute of Bioethics

---

[1] The Agreement on Trade-Related Aspects of Intellectual Property Rights (TRIPS), a basic document adopted in 1994 by the World Trade Organization (WTO), establishes obligations of Member Nations to enforce patents and other intellectual property rights. The TRIPS Agreement permits "compulsory licensing", which is "authorization, given by a government, to use a patented invention without the consent of the patent-holder" upon payment of a small royalty, in order to allow a country to provide treatments that would otherwise be unavailable because of the patent. For more information, visit http://www.wto.org/english/tratop_e/trips_e/t_agm1_e.htm (accessed 25 August 2008).

Case 19

Pneumonia vaccine trial

A childhood vaccine for pneumococcal disease, one of the most important causes of child deaths in the developing world, has been developed by a European pharmaceutical company and tested at a site in Africa. The goal of the trial was to determine how many children would be protected from the disease before the age of 3 years. In this community, and in the region overall, approximately 90% of the childhood deaths caused by pneumococcal disease occur in children younger than 3 years.

After community consultation and extensive efforts to obtain meaningful informed consent, 20 000 infants were enrolled in the vaccine trial. Participants were randomized and half received the trial vaccine. After 3 years, 90% of those who were vaccinated remained free of the disease. Those in the control group had infection and mortality rates comparable to those that prevailed in recent years in this population.

Ordinarily, vaccines and other interventions which are proven effective in a randomized placebo-controlled trial are offered to all participants in the control group soon after the conclusion of the trial. Some of the scientists in this study, however, became reluctant to follow that practice in this trial. Their concern was that the study provided a unique opportunity to determine whether the vaccine protected children who were older than 3 years; if the controls were vaccinated at the conclusion of the trial, an ongoing study in older children would have no controls. The same considerations applied to longer-term monitoring of adverse post-trial events. Both of these issues – protection of children older than 3 years, and long-term safety – might play a role in determining whether the vaccine would be widely used in the future, and many children's lives might depend on the result. Moreover, if (as turned out to be the case) the results of the first trial were definitive for children aged 3 years and younger, it might be impossible to conduct any further controlled trial of the vaccine. This was, in the view of these scientists, a unique opportunity. Their concerns, however, were not incorporated into the study design, and all controls received the vaccine at the conclusion of the trial.

Questions

1 Were the dissenting scientists correct to urge that controls should not be vaccinated? If the parents had agreed to this condition in the informed consent, would this justify not vaccinating the control group at the conclusion of the study?

2 If the randomized, placebo-controlled trial design was justified, why would it be unjustified to decline to vaccinate the controls?

3 Would any further test of the effect of these vaccines on children older than 3 years, and of long-term safety, be justified?

Case 20

Early termination of a trial

From a global perspective, breast cancer is the most common cause of cancer deaths in women. Although breast cancer is increasingly being discovered early enough for surgery to be a beneficial intervention, many surviving women live in fear of recurrence. The search for interventions to prevent this eventuality has for many years been a high priority for oncologists.

A promising drug was tested in a randomized control trial for women who had obtained maximum protection from other interventions. After enrolment of the designated number of participants, investigators intended to continue the trial until a statistically significant difference in outcomes was established between the test and control groups, or 5 years had passed, whichever came first. A data safety monitoring board was formed. Its members – scientists who had no other links to the experiment – would be given periodic reports of adverse events and other safety data, and would monitor trends.

No significant difference in outcomes had been established between the two groups after three years of the study, but a trend was emerging that was strongly in favour of the treatment group. The data safety monitoring board recommended that the trial should be stopped and that all participants be offered the new drug. The investigators accepted their recommendation, reasoning that further withholding of the experimental intervention from the women in the control group could not be justified.

To their surprise, the investigators were criticized by a leading breast-cancer organization, which represented women with breast cancer and their families. The organization's concern was that by stopping the trial before the agreed statistically significant end-points had been reached, the trial's results remained uncertain. Whether the trend represented a real benefit of the drug would now be impossible to determine; moreover, it would be difficult or impossible to receive approval for a second study of the same drug. Clinicians worldwide would be very likely to offer the drug to women after surgery for breast cancer to prevent recurrence, either in combination with or after other forms of treatment. With doubt remaining about the effectiveness of the drug, these women might endure the drug's side-effects and bear its cost without receiving any benefit. Comments from other sources were divided.

Questions

1. Given that the trial design had not called for early termination in the case of a strong trend that was short of statistical significance, should the board have issued an opinion to the investigators on the basis of the trend?

2. Should the REC have been involved in this decision making and the final recommendations to the investigators?

3. Should DSMBs be restricted to alerting investigators to serious adverse events, except for announcing that agreed endpoints have been reached?

4. "Statistical significance" is considered an objective measure of truth in scientific outcome data. In what situations may investigators choose to ignore this and make "moral choices". What conditions must be satisfied before moral choices are allowed to over-rule scientific methods? In this situation, if the investigators had ignored the recommendation of the DSMB, could they have justified their action to women in the control group who suffered a recurrence of breast cancer before the trial was terminated?

Case 21

Pregnancy in health research

Researchers from an international non-governmental organization based in North America receive a grant to test a vaginal microbicide for its ability to prevent new HIV infections.[1] The ideal study location would allow researchers to recruit a large number of women who were HIV-negative but who were at exceptionally high risk for contracting HIV. Many of the study participants, therefore, might be commercial sex workers in a country with a high prevalence of HIV. After some investigation into potential research locations, the researchers decide that the multi-site study should be conducted in four African and one South Asian country.

The drug being tested has not yet undergone any Segment III preclinical studies and so cannot clearly be used safely by pregnant women. Thus, the study protocol clearly states that pregnancy or a desire to become pregnant during the coming year precludes study participation. This exclusion criterion is carefully implemented during study recruitment. In accordance with recommended research practice,[2] HIV prevention and contraceptive counselling will be provided. Study investigators will also conduct monthly pregnancy testing to ensure that any woman who becomes pregnant during the study suspends her participation until she is no longer pregnant. The informed consent reiterates that the contraceptive effect of the study drug is unknown, and that if a woman becomes pregnant while participating in the study she should cease use of the drug immediately and end her participation until she is no longer pregnant.

A few months after the study commences, researchers notice that many women are suspending study participation because they are getting pregnant. After further investigation, researchers document that the average time that women are not participating in the study due to pregnancy is just less than 3 months. Thus, many of the women who become pregnant seem to be having either spontaneous or induced abortions and then rejoining the study.

In the countries participating in the study, abortion on request during the first trimester of pregnancy is permitted in only two countries, A and B; however, for several reasons, safe abortions remains unavailable for many women in both these countries. In country C, abortion is allowed for multiple health indications, including preservation of the mental health of the woman, but abortion on request is not legally permitted. Also in country C, women can struggle to find providers willing to do abortions on mental-health grounds, and the cost of such procedures is usually quite high. In countries D and E, legal abortion is available only to save the life of the woman; however, both safe and unsafe services exist at a price.

Questions

1. What should the researchers do now that they know many participants are becoming pregnant while participating in the study and that many are probably having illegal and perhaps unsafe abortions?

2. Should the study sponsors provide safe abortions to women who inadvertently become pregnant while participating in the study?

3. What if a donor prohibits recipients of grants from providing any information or services related to abortion?

4. Should the study investigators warn prospective participants that unwanted pregnancy is a study risk, that abortion in their country is not available (or not widely available) on request; and that unsafe abortion presents a great risk to a woman's health and life?

5. With the knowledge that we have now, should such studies ever be done in countries in which safe abortion on request is not legally and readily available?

6. Under what circumstances would you be comfortable about conducting such a study in the countries listed? What about in other countries?

Adapted from a case study contributed by Dr Brooke Ronald Johnson, World Health Organization

---

[1] Vaginal microbicides are chemical agents used topically by women within the vagina in order to prevent infection by HIV and potentially by other enveloped viruses and sexually transmitted pathogens. Prototype microbicides are designed to be inserted prior to sexual intercourse and could also be contraceptive, although most current potential microbicides are not.(Weber J, Desai K, Darbyshire J, on behalf of the Microbicides Development Programme (2005) The Development of Vaginal Microbicides for the Prevention of HIV Transmission. PLoS Med 2(5): e142 doi:10.1371/journal.pmed.0020142). The development of vaginal microbicide assumes great significance in the context of the HIV epidemic, because an effective microbicide would be an effective women-controlled method. Condoms, though very effective against the transmission of HIV remain under the control of the male partner.

[2] See for example, UNAIDS/WHO. Ethical Considerations in Biomedical HIV Prevention Trials – UNAIDS/WHO guidance document. Geneva: Joint United Nations Programme on HIV/AIDS (UNAIDS) and the World Health Organization, 2007. http://data.unaids.org/pub/Report/2007/jc1399-ethicalconsiderations_en.pdf (accessed 4 September 2008)

Case 22

Acting in the face of conflicting evidence

> Although this case is based on research and a situation that happened in the mid-1990s, it is included here because the ethical questions remain relevant. See Case 34 for more details on the quinacrine trials.

Effective and accessible methods of avoiding pregnancy are important not only for control of family size but also for reduction of maternal mortality, which has been estimated at over half a million deaths per year, most of which are in developing countries. Since surgical sterilization is not readily available in many low-resource countries, alternative, non-surgical methods have been sought.

Since the first trials in the 1960s, the non-surgical permanent method that has received the most attention is intrauterine application of quinacrine hydrochloride.[1] Over the course of several decades, approximately 104 500 women in more than 20 countries (mostly in Asia) were sterilized by this method. In 1990, however, there were reports of an apparently increased rate of cancer in a group of 600 South American women who had had quinacrine sterilizations. These reports, along with laboratory studies in North America and elsewhere indicating that the drug caused cells to mutate in vitro, led to the suspension of the major programme in which quinacrine had been provided worldwide for sterilization.

Despite the controversy about this use of quinacrine, a small group of North American scientists affiliated with an institute for population research continued to champion the product. They argued that quinacrine was nearly as effective as surgical sterilization (95-98% effective in prevention of pregnancy *vs* 99% for surgery) and much safer (two deaths per 100 000 women surgically sterilized in the United States of America, but no deaths reported in the more than 100 000 cases of quinacrine sterilization). Further, they cited data from one of the countries which had been using the drug for sterilizations that showed 7.6 maternal deaths avoided for every 1000 sterilizations.

The scientists from the population-research institute contended that the potential benefits of non-surgical sterilization were indisputable. Conversely, they argued that no association between quinacrine sterilization and future increased risk of cancer could be ascertained on the basis of the small South American sample studied. They also noted that any cancer risk associated with the method must be negligible or non-existent since no increase in cancer incidence had been recorded in the millions of people who have taken the drug orally over the past 60 years for parasitic diseases.

The proponents mobilized a network of doctors, nurses, and midwives to administer quinacrine, which was obtained from a European manufacturer at no cost, for the purpose of sterilization. Even though quinacrine had never been approved for sterilization, they did not propose to conduct further studies; when quinacrine was criticized in 1990, some women's advocacy groups labelled the quinacrine studies as unethical experimentation on poor women. Instead, the institute scientists aimed to implement programmes to provide quinacrine for female sterilization, on that ground that denying women access to a safe, inexpensive, and easily administered form of sterilization would be immoral.

---

[1] A drug which is administered orally to treat certain worm infections in humans and which had been previously used to treat malaria. In the 1960s, researchers began exploring quinacrine as a sclerosing agent to cause scar tissue in the fallopian tubes. In the late 1970s, the drug was formulated into pellets for insertion through the cervix using a modified intrauterine device (IUD) inserter or similar apparatus.

Questions

1. If quinacrine is the cause of the cancer cluster in the South American country where the trial took place, can use of the drug still be justified in settings where maternal mortality is high, and access to methods of contraception and safe surgical sterilization is poor?

2. What is the relation between the balance of harm and benefit in the design of a clinical trial and the balance of harm and benefit in the clinical use of a drug for an unapproved use?

3. Should the export of a drug to developing countries be allowed when this drug is not registered in the exporting country? What about when it is registered but its use is not the "standard of care" in the exporting country?

4. Would you consider the action of the scientists from the population-research institute to be a type of "misconduct"? What role does the scientific community have in regulation of misconduct of its members?

Chapter IV

Voluntary Informed Consent

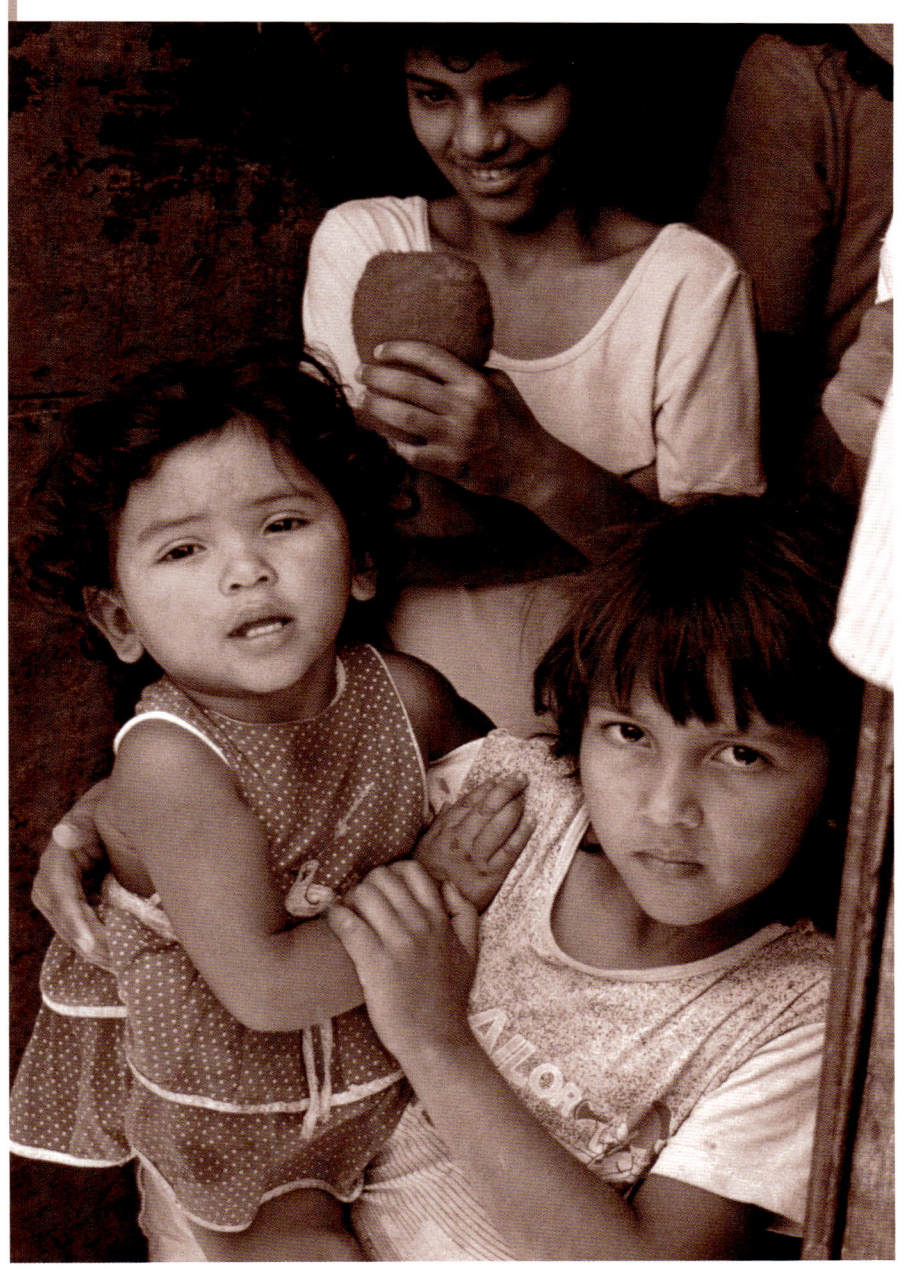

© WHO

Introduction: Chapter IV

Is consent to research voluntary, knowing, and competent?

Although informed consent had appeared in codes of ethics for scientific research as early as the nineteenth century,[1] its central importance was firmly established in the "Doctors' Trial" before the Nuremberg Tribunal at the end of the Second World War. In passing judgment on the Nazi doctors, the court articulated a set of principles for ethical research with human beings. This ten-point statement of ethical imperatives for researchers, which became known as the *Nuremberg Code*,[2] provided the groundwork on which subsequent statements of research ethics, such as the World Medical Association's *Declaration of Helsinki*[3] (first issued in 1964) and the Council for International Organizations of Medical Sciences' (CIOMS) *International Ethical Guidelines for Biomedical Research Involving Human Subjects* (first published in 1993),[4] have elaborated. While researchers and research ethics committees refer to the more recent guidance (updated versions of the *Declaration of Helsinki* and the CIOMS *International Ethical Guidelines)*, rather than to the Nuremberg Code, it is, nevertheless, still useful to reflect on the origins of informed consent.

The first principle in the *Nuremberg Code* is so important that it deserves to be set forth in full:

> The voluntary consent of the human subject is absolutely essential.
>
> This means that the person involved should have legal capacity to give consent; should be so situated as to be able to exercise free power of choice, without the intervention of any element of force, fraud, deceit, duress, over-reaching, or other ulterior form of constraint or coercion; and should have sufficient knowledge and comprehension of the elements of the subject matter involved, as to enable him to make an understanding and enlightened decision. This latter element requires that, before the acceptance of an affirmative decision by the experimental subject, there should be made known to him the nature, duration, and purpose of the experiment; the method and means by which it is to be conducted; all inconveniences and hazards reasonably to be expected; and the effects upon his health or person, which may possibly come from his participation in the experiment.

The duty and responsibility for ascertaining the quality of the consent rests upon each individual who initiates, directs or engages in the experiment. It is a personal duty and responsibility which may not be readily delegated to another. The Nuremberg Tribunal's placement of this provision at the top of the list of principles indicates its primacy: without consent by the individual research participant, no experimentation may proceed. Consent, in this view, is where research ethics begins.

Three essential elements

The Code's first principle emphasizes three essential qualities of valid consent:

- the person must have the capacity to give consent;
- the person must be acting voluntarily; and
- the person must have been provided with sufficient comprehensible information to make an enlightened decision.

---

[1] Vollman J, Winau R. Informed Consent in Human Experimentation Before the Nuremberg Code. *BMJ*, 1996; 313:1445-1447.
http://www.bmj.com/archive/7070nd1.htm (accessed 10 April 2008)

[2] Nuremberg Code. In: Trials of War Criminals Before the Nuremberg Military Tribunals Under Control Council Law No. 10, Vol. 2, Nuremberg, October 1946-April 1949. Permissible Medical Experiments on Human Subjects. Washington: United States Government Printing Office (2), 1949:181-182.
http://www.hhs.gov/ohrp/references/nurcode.htm (accessed 28 August 2008)

[3] World Medical Association. *Declaration of Helsinki: Ethical Principles for Medical Research Involving Human Subjects*. Helsinki, Finland: WMA, 1964. Revised and updated version 2008. http://www.wma.net/e/policy/b3.htm (accessed 5 June 2009)

[4] Council for International Organizations of Medical Sciences (CIOMS). International Ethical Guidelines for Biomedical Research Involving Human Subjects. Geneva, Switzerland: Council for International Organizations of Medical Sciences (CIOMS), 2002. http://www.cioms.ch/frame_guidelines_nov_2002.htm (accessed 10 April 2008)

Capacity to give consent

The phrase "capacity to give consent" has two dimensions – firstly, that individuals are legally empowered to make their own decisions, and secondly, that they have the capacity to understand and question the information on which they base their decisions. The first dimension of this capacity is often taken for granted when dealing with adults, who are presumed to be legally competent. The second dimension is often ignored in the context of health research. Research often involves terminology, methods, and assumptions that are unfamiliar to those who do not work in that area under study, and which are likely to be alien to potential participants who live in places where research is not a routine or familiar activity. How do adults who are competent in all other respects make competent decisions about participating in activities which involve methods or assumptions that are unfamiliar (and often incomprehensible) to them? On the other hand, the assumption that those who are not legally competent *should not* give consent is under-inclusive because it ignores the capacity of some minors to make competent decisions.

Voluntariness

The voluntariness element was examined in detail by the Nuremberg judges because of the circumstances in which the Code was prepared – namely the trial of doctors who had performed inhumane experiments on concentration camp inmates from whom any supposed consent was plainly coerced. In order to avoid coercion in any contemporary contexts, the requirement of voluntariness remains essential. It can, however, be overlooked – or even assumed – because investigators themselves might not be aware that even though they do not use force, duress, or other forms of overt coercion, the potential participant might feel that they have little choice as to whether to participate or not. Investigators (and the RECs that review their protocols) should, nonetheless, be sensitive to circumstances that can severely constrain participants' sense of freedom of choice, such as offers of money, gifts, or free medical care to people who may not otherwise have access to it. Such offers are not literally coercive, since prospective participants are at liberty to decline them. At the same time, they might feel compelled to accept any offerings made by the investigator because it might be the only way to obtain food or medical care for themselves and their families.

Another aspect of the voluntariness requirement concerns research that involves the potential participant's physician or health care worker. Patients have a very specific trust-based relationship with their physicians and other health care workers, which is grounded in the understanding that they, as patients, will receive the care that is best for them. When the physician or health care worker changes roles from therapeutic helper to researcher and recruiter of participants, two challenges to voluntariness can occur. Firstly, the patient might not fully comprehend the conflict of missions between treatment (arising from a doctor-patient relationship in which the patient's interests take priority) and research (arising from an investigator-participant relationship where the aim is the generation of new knowledge). The second challenge is that the patient might feel that he/she must agree to participate, or face repercussions. To ensure voluntariness, a new "contract" needs to be entered into, and the informed consent fulfils this purpose.

The voluntariness of informed consent has been less explored in bioethics literature than the element of disclosure (or comprehension), possibly because of its abstract nature. For this and other reasons, RECs often face great difficulty in interpreting and applying the requirement of voluntariness. Too severe a limitation could result either in excluding research on conditions that primarily affect poor populations or in restricting the ability of investigators to provide health services that might be scientifically necessary for their studies, out of concern that such services may be seen to be "undue inducements" for participants. When it appears that some participants' consent cannot be counted as fully voluntary – at least not in the way that a wealthier volunteer's participation would be – the REC might conclude that the study should not be approved; decide that it should be conducted in another population that is less constrained by circumstances; or approve the study after weighing the concerns about voluntariness against other ethical objectives.

Provision of sufficient and comprehensible information

Most discussion of informed consent has focused on the information element: what needs to be disclosed and how this should be done in order to enable potential participants to make "an understood and enlightened decision". The broad consensus is that RECs should expect investigators to provide:

- a full account of anticipated and potential risks and benefits and, where relevant, a comparison to alternative treatments;
- a clear statement of the purpose of the research;
- the names of the study sponsors;
- a declaration of any potentially conflicting interest on the part of the investigators; and
- an account of the care and compensation that participants would receive if any adverse events or other injuries occurred.

These must be disclosed in a written consent form or by an oral equivalent for participants who are illiterate or in settings where a written form is judged to be inappropriate. But information is not in itself sufficient to ensure the informed participation of the individual; he or she must not only be told but must also be in a position to understand what is told. In studies of a complex nature that also involve considerable risks, investigators also have an obligation to formally assess how well the research participants have understood the information provided to them.[1]

The functions of consent

If informed consent by each individual research participant were an absolute requirement that could be fulfilled with a universal or completely standardized form and process, ethical review would be much easier. Research ethics committees would simply need to ensure that the form had certain specified information and that it would be signed by the participant.[2] In practice, however, a process or document that is suitable for ensuring informed consent in one situation might be completely inappropriate in another. The type of informed consent process that is appropriate depends on the reason for the requirement of informed consent in a specific context, whether it is to assure self-determination and autonomy; to protect people from unacceptable harm; or to transfer responsibility from investigators to participants.

---

[1] CIOMS. Commentary on Guideline 4. In: *International Ethical Guidelines for Biomedical Research Involving Human Subjects*. Geneva, Switzerland: Council for International Organizations of Medical Sciences, 2002. http://www.cioms.ch/frame_guidelines_nov_2002.htm (accessed 10 April 08)

[2] Lindegger G, et al. Beyond the checklist. Assessing Understanding for HIV Vaccine Trial Participation in South Africa. *Journal of Acquired Immune Deficiency Syndrome*, 2006; 43:5. http://www.saavi.org.za/beyond.pdf (accessed 10 April 2008)

Assurance of self-determination and autonomy: Insistence on informed consent gives the individual the opportunity and the right to receive full information and to say "no", and acknowledges that the person's wishes and agreement are sovereign. Those who may choose for themselves on matters of personal significance are often those who enjoy the highest status in a community: the existence of a requirement for competent consent serves as a reminder that everyone, irrespective of their community status, has the right to speak for themselves. (In the case of a young child or mentally incompetent person, they have the right to have someone act in their best interests.) On occasion, individuals offer, or are asked to volunteer to accept risks or discomfort purely for the benefit of others or the furtherance of knowledge. An individual's willingness to volunteer does not excuse the scientist from striving to reduce risks to the fullest possible extent, and the REC is not required to approve such research even if individuals have agreed to accept those risks. But individuals who are not competent to give consent cannot volunteer in this way, and should not be asked to do so; for them, risk without compensating direct benefit is much harder to justify.

Protection: Barring coercion, most people will not participate in research that poses serious harms without compensating individual or, perhaps, community benefit. The full disclosure of risks required in the informed consent process thus allows people to protect themselves from harms that exceed, in likelihood or degree, those they are willing to accept, whether for their own benefit or to serve science.

Transfer of responsibility: Even when consent has been obtained, investigators remain responsible for participants' health, safety, and well-being. Nevertheless, consent does effect some transfer of responsibility from the investigators to participants. If risks are fully disclosed, and the REC finds that participants' exposure to risk is justified by the benefits (to participants and to others), the research may proceed. The REC, however, must judge whether a research project proposes to assign responsibility appropriately – both for any discomfort, pain, and adverse outcomes that are known in advance and for any that might arise unexpectedly – based on what has been agreed upon in advance.

Dilemmas in applying principles of informed consent

The primacy of consent in research ethics has not been seriously challenged since Nuremberg. Nevertheless, the Code's unambiguous and emphatic requirement of individual, voluntary informed consent by competent participants doesn't provide sufficient guidance for ethical dilemmas that often arise today in research with human participants. More recent guidelines, such as the *Declaration of Helsinki* and the CIOMS *International Ethical Guidelines for Biomedical Research Involving Human Subjects* have been more flexible and inclusive, without losing sight of the purposes of informed consent and a meaningful process of informed consent. Strict principles of informed consent can be difficult to apply if participants are incapable of consent; if the research requires deception; if the research has low risks and individual consent would be impractical or costly to obtain; if participants prefer to delegate the right to informed consent; or if the participants do not have the right to say no.

Some participants are incapable of consent: Taken literally, the Code forbids experimentation with young children and with others who lack the capacity to consent. The price to be paid for such scruples has been also borne by the same groups, for until recently, for example, new drugs and medicines were never tested on children; instead, results of the research done on adults was extrapolated to the paediatric population, in the expectation that children would react the same. However, it is now understood that children are not miniature adults, and drugs can often act differently in this group. It is now considered unethical to exclude children from participation in research that is pertinent to their needs and care.

Instead of barring research in those who lack the capacity to consent, recent guidelines have addressed the issue by specifying who can serve as a "surrogate" decision-maker; what additional issues need to be considered; and what safeguards must be put in place, including the importance of assessing the risk-benefit ratio in this group. A restrictive interpretation of this guideline would require that research must aim to provide a net benefit for participants, whereas an alternative interpretation would permit research that imposes only minor risks, on the condition that the research could potentially produce substantial benefits and could not be conducted with an alternative cohort of participants who are capable of giving their own consent (for example, adults instead of children). A similar problem arises in clinical trials of new treatments for conditions that need rapid emergency treatment while patients are still temporarily incapacitated; regulations in some countries now allow research to be conducted without prior consent or surrogate permission once the research has been vetted and approved by groups in the community where it will be undertaken.

Some study designs require deception: In order to avoid bias, a research design sometimes requires that participants should not know the nature of the research project. They are, in this sense, deceived, since they have not been fully apprised of the purpose and methods of the research nor given the opportunity to provide or withhold their informed consent. Such a design is not acceptable in most research, and, for example, never in a clinical drug trial but it is not uncommon in some social science based health research. (A study design which requires deception should not be confused with a study which simply deceives because it does not provide the information that it should provide.)

In general, designs that involve deception are of two types – researchers might either need to withhold information, or might need to give misleading information in order to avoid biasing participants' responses. For example, in Case Study 7 in Chapter II on *Issues in Study Design*, in order to find out if local drug sellers are prescribing and selling appropriate medicine to treat childhood diarrhoea, research assistants pose as customers and request diarrhoeal medicine from local drug sellers. The sellers do not know that they are part of a research study which they have not consented to and have been misled into believing that the medication is for real children. Since the *Nuremberg Code*'s prohibition of "fraud" requires researchers to tell the truth, this would seem to be an unacceptable study design. Would the study be more permissible if the drug sellers had a full "debriefing" (consisting of disclosure and explanation of the deception) after their interaction with the research assistants? The CIOMS *Guidelines* give some guidance on how to deal with research studies that need to withhold information or practise deception and they require ethics committees to judge whether or not such research should be conducted, or whether the study design should be changed.

In some low risk research individual consent would be impractical or very costly to obtain: Should there be a uniform standard for informed consent in all types of research, ranging from complex clinical trials to population-scale epidemiological studies that pose little or no risk to human participants? Insisting on informed consent in some zero-risk studies might mislead participants into thinking that their health and safety are at risk. Obtaining consent in studies involving large populations can also be extremely impractical and costly. Another important example in health-related research concerns tissue donated for one study which a researcher a decade later would like to use for another similar study that had not been anticipated when the tissue was initially collected and stored. Assuming that the original consent did not encompass the second study, must informed consent be obtained again? Or, since re-contacting the participants would be difficult – and for some impossible given the passage of time – would it ever be reasonable to conclude that anyone who consented to the first study would also consent to the second, or that participants' interest in giving consent is outweighed by the value of the study?

Some participants prefer to delegate their rights to informed consent. The *Nuremberg Code* specifically states that informed consent "may not be delegated to another…" The context of this statement in the *Code* was that concentration camp prisoners had not been allowed to exercise their right to decide for themselves whether or not to participate in research. For cultural or personal reasons, some individuals want decisions about their participation in research to be made by others, such as their family or the family's elders. Such proxy decision-making is accepted by physicians when seeking consent for treatment. Under what circumstances, if any, is it appropriate when a consent is sought for research to allow potential participants to delegate this decision to a proxy? Should people who do not want to consent for themselves not be recruited because they were unwilling to engage in the informed consent process directly? In the context of research conducted in a defined population, may a duly elected community leader consent for an entire community; if so, can they decide for all studies or only for certain types? What about a traditional leader, such as a tribal chief or village elder? The *Declaration of Helsinki* and the CIOMS *International Ethical Guidelines for Biomedical Research Involving Human Subjects* are clear that, for biomedical research, individual consent is still required and cannot be delegated, although consultation with others is very acceptable and sometimes essential.

Some participants do not have the right to say no. Not every person being studied may, in fact, have the right to refuse. For example, a literal interpretation of the *Nuremberg Code* would require biographers to ask the consent of their subjects before undertaking research; such a requirement would chill historical investigation and shield public figures from scrutiny. Beyond extreme cases in historical research, opinion remains divided about other social science studies, from linguistics to ethnomusicology. Even in medical research, part of the task of the REC is to determine which parties to a research project have the right to refuse to participate. For example, an investigator adhering to the WHO guidelines for research on domestic violence against women would fully inform female participants of the study's aims and risks but would not inform their husbands of the specific nature of the study or seek their consent.

Consent as a process

Informed consent should not be seen as a one-time activity. It is a process that is often initiated even before the research protocol is written up. Community consultations on whether or not a research study should be carried out in that population should begin at the planning stage of the research. Once the protocol is written and accepted by scientific and ethical review committees, the consent process may involve community meetings in which the research project is explained, and questions are answered. Often potential participants need time to consult other family members or friends, and the signing of an informed consent is only the last step in that process. Traditionally, the signed informed consent may be seen as the most vital step, but a progressive ethics committee will give equal weight (if not more weight) to the process of obtaining consent. Finally, subsequent changes in the study may require that re-consent be obtained and, in some very complex, high risk research studies, consent might need to be renewed at each follow-up visit, with emphasis on the freedom to withdraw at any stage without penalty, and addressing any concerns that the participants might have.

When is the requirement of informed consent satisfied?

Regulations about informed consent often include checklists of points that investigators and RECs ought to consider; the *CIOMS Guidelines*, for example, list 26 elements that should presumptively be included in every consent form. Yet a REC that must assess whether the requirement of informed consent has been met might often need to make subtle moral judgments rather than simply check off items on a list. In the most straightforward cases, the REC must determine whether all risks, benefits, alternatives, and other essential information have been disclosed in a way that ensures that prospective participants can fully understand what is being asked of them, and decide freely whether to give their consent. However, as previously discussed, some study designs might require full disclosure to be compromised, and some research participants might be in circumstances or have mental barriers that constrain their ability to make voluntary choices.

A REC faced with such complex circumstances might do well to first identify the purposes or functions of informed consent in the context of the proposal. Should the ideal of complete disclosure and voluntary participation by fully competent participants not be feasible, what alternative mechanisms could achieve these aims? Though all RECs would agree with the Nuremberg Tribunal that the Nazi experiments on unconsenting victims were a travesty of justice and morality, there is some room for reasoned disagreement on some of the complex and nuanced ethical dilemmas involving informed consent that are presented by contemporary research protocols.

Suggested readings

Bhutta ZA. Beyond Informed Consent. *Bulletin of the World Health Organization*, 2004, 82:771-777.

"Although a relatively recent phenomenon, the role of informed consent in human research is central to its ethical regulation and conduct. However, guidelines often recommend procedures for obtaining informed consent (usually written consent) that are difficult to implement in developing countries. This paper reviews the guidelines for obtaining informed consent and also discusses prevailing views on current controversies, ambiguities and problems with these guidelines and suggests potential solutions."

http://www.who.int/bulletin/volumes/82/10/771.pdf
(accessed 10 May 2008)

Henderson GE, et al. Clinical Trials and Medical Care: Defining the Therapeutic Misconception. *PLoS Medicine*, 2007; 4(11): e324.

"A key component of informed consent to participate in medical research is the understanding that research is not the same as treatment. However, studies have found that some research participants do not appreciate important differences between research and treatment, a phenomenon called "therapeutic misconception." A consistent definition of therapeutic misconception is missing from the literature, and this hinders attempts to define its prevalence or ways to reduce it. This paper proposes a new definition and describes how it can be operationalized."

http://dx.doi.org/10.1371/journal.pmed.0040324
(accessed 25 August 2008)

Lindegger G, Richter LM. HIV Vaccine Trials: Critical Issues in Informed Consent. *South African Journal of Science*, 2000;96:313-317.

"Informed consent (IC), a fundamental principle of ethics in medical research, is recognized as a vital component of HIV vaccine trials. There are different notions of IC, some legally based and others based on ethics. It is argued that, though legal indemnity is necessary, vaccine trials should be founded on fully ethical considerations." This article explores the differences between the legal and moral arguments for obtaining informed consent from research participants and examines the implications of each before ultimately deciding in favour of a moral or ethical rationale.

http://www.saavi.org.za/lindegger.pdf
(accessed 9 May 2008)

Marshall PA. Ethical Challenges in Study Design and Informed Consent for Health Research in Resource-poor Settings. Geneva, Switzerland: WHO/TDR, 2007.

"This review considers ethical challenges to research design and informed consent in biomedical and behavioural studies conducted in resource-poor settings. A review of the literature explores relevant social, cultural, and ethical issues in the conduct of biomedical and social health research in developing countries. Ten case vignettes illustrate ethical challenges that arise in international research with culturally diverse populations" In addition, this publication offers recommendations to researchers and policy-makers concerned with ethical practices in multinational studies conducted in resource-poor settings. Issues of community consultation, decisional authority to consent, and power inequities are addressed in the context of consent.

https://www.who.int/tdr/publications/tdr-research-publications/ethical-challenges-study-design/pdf/ethical_challenges.pdf
(accessed 30 August 2008)

Molyneux CS, et al. 'Even If They Ask You To Stand By A Tree All Day, You Will Have To Do It (Laughter)…!': Community Voices on the Notion and Practice of Informed Consent for Biomedical Research in Developing Countries. *Social Science and Medicine*, 2005; 61:443-54.

"Ethical dilemmas in biomedical research, especially in vulnerable populations, often spark heated debate. Despite recommendations and guidelines, many issues remain controversial, including the relevance, prioritisation and application of individual voluntary informed consent in non-Western settings. The voices of the people likely to be the subjects of research have been notably absent from the debate." The authors share their findings from discussions with groups of community members living in the rural study area of a large research unit in Kenya. They emphasize that the failure to appreciate the spectrum of views and understandings held by community members risks researchers responding inadequately to the needs and values of those on whom the success of most biomedical research depends.

http://dx.doi.org/10.1016/j.socscimed.2004.12.003
(accessed 25 August 2008)

Préziosi M, et al. Practical Experiences in Obtaining Informed Consent for a Vaccine Trial in Rural Africa. *New England Journal of Medicine*, 1997;336:370-373.

"There is considerable debate about the appropriateness of obtaining individual informed consent in non-Western cultures. In the process of conducting a study of a new pertussis vaccine in a rural community in Senegal, we sought to evaluate the incorporation of clear procedures for obtaining individual informed consent from parents. In this part of Senegal, consent for all previous research with human subjects had been obtained from community leaders on behalf of all eligible members of the community. Individuals could subsequently decline to participate."

http://content.nejm.org/cgi/content/extract/336/5/370
(accessed 25 August 2008)

Rotini C, et al. Community Engagement and Informed Consent in the International Hapmap Project. *Community Genetics*, 2007;10:186-198.

"The International HapMap Consortium has developed the HapMap, a resource that describes the common patterns of human genetic variation (haplotypes). Processes of community/public consultation and individual informed consent were implemented in each locality where samples were collected to understand and attempt to address both individual and group concerns". The experience of approaching genetic variation research in a spirit of openness was a positive one and the authors suggest that this openness can help investigators to "better appreciate the views of the communities whose samples they seek to study and help communities become more engaged in the science."

http://dx.doi.org/10.1159/000101761
(accessed 25 August 2008)

Case 23

Testing high doses of vitamin A on children

The ministry of health of a West African country receives a grant from a foreign medical institute to collaborate with its investigators on a double-blind study designed to assess the effect of periodic high doses of vitamin A on the incidences of childhood diarrhoea and acute respiratory infections (ARI). High-dose vitamin A capsules or placebo would be administered in a double-blind fashion every 4 months for 1 year to children from 6 months to 5 years. A record of morbidity (diarrhoea and ARI) and mortality data would be measured biweekly and blood samples would be drawn (less than 2cc) at 0, 6, and 12 months to test vitamin A status. The daily affairs of this traditional, rural community are governed by a traditional leader and council of elders but the national government retains control of other municipal affairs, including tax collection, the police, and the military.

The chief and council call a meeting to inform the community of the proposed study. In a festive environment, the investigators describe the study and answer all questions from members of the community (men, women, and children) and from the council. After a brief meeting, the village chief and council give their approval. Shortly thereafter, in accordance with the guidelines provided by the research ethics committee at the foreign investigators' institution, the field staff begin to go from house to house to obtain parents' signatures on the informed consent forms that are necessary to allow their children to participate in the study. The parents, however, say that since the chief has already approved of the study they do not need to sign anything. They also explain to the researchers that they usually do not sign anything because they cannot read what they are signing.

On the second day, the field team making the home visits is summoned to the chief's house where they are politely informed that their seeking individual signatures is both unnecessary and insulting. The fact that the chief and council has approved is enough. When the field staff explain that they are required by the grant agreement to obtain signed informed consent forms, they are told that if they insist on doing so they will have to leave the community.

Questions

1. Is individual informed consent a culturally bound concept (from developed countries) or is it a universal principle that ought not be compromised?

2. May the chief and the council provide informed consent for the community? Should they?

3. How crucial is individual informed consent in this setting?

4. Are there circumstances when individual informed consent is unnecessary?

5. Is the purpose of informed consent to protect the participant and/or the investigator?

6. How should the field team handle this problem? What should the granting institution do?

Case 24

Breast cancer in South Asia

> This case is based on research that was conducted at a time when the role of tamoxifen for management of breast cancer was not well defined. Currently, it is an accepted form of adjuvant therapy in these patients.

Researchers from a North American university propose to study a new adjuvant therapy[1] called tamoxifen[2] for the treatment of breast cancer in premenopausal women in a South Asian country. In the United States of America, the standard treatment for any stage of breast cancer for this demographic is surgery followed by some form of adjuvant therapy, such as radiation, chemotherapy, or hormonal treatments. The researchers contend that a placebo-controlled trial in the United States of America would not be possible because adjuvant treatment is widely accepted there and patients are unwilling to accept anything less than the standard regimen.

In the Asian country, however, adjuvant treatments are only occasionally used largely because of limited resources. When they are used, it is often in ways that are unlikely to benefit to the patient. The researchers, therefore, anticipate no difficulty in enrolling 350 premenopausal women with operable breast cancer in a randomized, controlled trial of surgical oophorectomy[3] and tamoxifen. Both groups will undergo surgical removal of the breast cancer before enrolment. The active group will then be treated with the anti-cancer drug tamoxifen after the surgical removal of both ovaries, while the control group will be observed but will not receive either adjuvant ovarian removal or tamoxifen. The researchers claim that if successful, removal of the ovaries followed by tamoxifen therapy will provide a more feasible alternative for low-income countries than will the long drawn out chemotherapy or radiotherapy that is the accepted adjuvant regimen in developed countries.

The principal investigator of the study considers waiving some elements of the informed consent process prescribed by standards in developed countries. In particular, she wants to omit anything that would oblige the treating doctor to express any uncertainty. This approach would mean that the treating doctor would not discuss alternative therapies with the patient; further, the random assignment of patients to proposed treatments would also have to be withheld.

The study's investigators claim that application of notions of informed consent from developed countries is impractical since they would be unacceptable to the country's physicians, political leaders, and most patients. The researchers contend that developed countries' standards of informed consent assume that doctors routinely encourage patients to participate in making decisions about their own care; conversely, in the study country paternalism prevails in health care and patients expect their physicians to tell them which treatment is appropriate. For a physician to openly express uncertainty about what is the best treatment would be unacceptable; in practice, when patients are given a choice between possible treatments they almost always choose the one that is recommended by their physician.

To document their claim about these cultural differences between the study country and the United States of America, the investigators presented the proposed study to several surrogate decision makers. These included:

- Four south asian immigrant women in the North American country where the university is located, two of their husbands, and one visiting PhD sociologist.

- The Vice President and the Chief of the International Relations Department of the South Asian country's Women's Union, both of whom have a PhD from an English language university.

- Physicians from the country that is involved in the study.

---

[1] Adjuvant therapies are designed to eradicate any microscopic deposits of cancer cells that have spread or metastasized from the primary breast cancer and have been demonstrated to increase women's chances of long-term survival. (For more information, see http://consensus.nih.gov/2000/2000AdjuvantTherapyBreastCancer114html.htm) accessed 26 August 2008

For updated information see http://www.nlm.nih.gov/medlineplus/ (accessed 26 August 2008).

[2] Tamoxifen, an anti-oestrogenic drug, has been used for almost two decades as the first-line endocrine therapy for postmenopausal women who have advanced metastatic breast cancer. Tamoxifen is also used as adjuvant therapy in patients with breast cancer and is being tested for use as a preventive agent. There is conclusive evidence that tamoxifen reduces the risk for contralateral breast cancer in women with a previous diagnosis of breast cancer.

[3] An oophorectomy involves the surgical removal of a woman's ovaries in order to greatly reduce production of the estrogen and progesterone hormones which, in premenopausal women contribute to both ovarian and breast cancers.

All the people consulted conclude that the proposed approach to the informed consent process is acceptable, and that to divulge the information about the randomization process to the women participating in the trial would be inappropriate.

Questions

1. Do differences between developed countries and the southern Asian country justify differences in approaches to informed consent in the context of this study?

2. Does the information that was gathered from the outside observers strengthen the case for the investigators' proposal about the process for obtaining informed consent? Why or why not?

3. Is it justified to do such a study in a resource-poor country because resource-rich countries will not tolerate any study that is seen to provide less than the highest standard of treatment?

Adapted from material developed for a workshop in Bangkok, Thailand, by the UNDP/UNFPA/WHO/World Bank Special Programme of Research, Development and Research Training in Human Reproduction.

Case 25

Testing a microbicide

Expansion of the range of woman-controlled methods to prevent all sexually transmitted infections (STIs) is critical to stemming the spread of the HIV/AIDS pandemic. A vaginal microbicide[1] could offer women the potential to protect themselves from HIV and other STIs. The ideal microbicide would be effective, safe, acceptable, affordable, colourless, odourless, tasteless, easy to store and use, and available in a variety of preparations. It should also be available in contraceptive and non-contraceptive formulations and obtainable without a prescription. However, since the first microbicide developed is unlikely to have all these characteristics, the immediate priority is to develop a microbicide that provides protection against STIs if used consistently by those who need it most, and that is safe.

Evidence suggests that microbicides are effective against many sexually transmitted pathogens when tested in the laboratory; they seem to be most effective when used by women as prophylaxis against cervical infection by the bacteria *Neisseria gonorrhoeae* and *Chlamydi trachomatis* and vaginal infection by *Trichomonas vaginalis*.[2] The protective benefits of microbicides for men have not been studied, although researchers believe that a woman's male partner would also be protected from infection by the woman's use of a vaginal microbicide.

At the time that the following study was designed, the prospects for the development of microbicides were promising. A consensus was growing among experts that development of a microbicide would be technically feasible. Many microbicide products were still undergoing phase I and II testing to establish their safety and toxicity levels.

Power to Women International (PWI), a North American non-profit research organization with a strongly feminist agenda, was planning a study of a microbicide in an African country. Laboratory tests had shown that the product blocked HIV attachment to target cells in vitro. Phase I testing of this product, in five countries, showed that the agent produced no clinically significant signs of irritation and that participants generally found it acceptable and easy to use. Since this was a phase I trial, however, these women used the product for only 10 days and were not sexually active during this time.

The PWI researchers designed a phase II trial with 300 participants to further assess the safety and efficacy of this product. This study was the first large-scale phase II microbicide trial in a population of women who were not sex workers, and the first to use a formulation that was not contraceptive. PWI conducted the study at two family planning clinics with co-investigators from a medical university in the host country. PWI funded renovations at each clinic to upgrade laboratory facilities and also covered the costs of hiring extra nursing and support staff for the study. Before the study commenced, the PWI researchers and representatives from the host-country university held meetings at the clinics to explain the study to potential participants and to elicit their feedback.

The study's inclusion criteria were that participants must be female, aged 18 years or older, HIV-negative at the time of enrolment, and be resident in the community for at least 1 year with no intention of leaving for 1 year after the start of the study. One of the researchers, with the aid of a translator, sought informed consent from every participant. Out of respect for the woman's autonomy, the researchers decided not to seek informed consent from their partners; women were neither encouraged to inform their partners of their involvement in the study, nor discouraged.

---

[1] Microbicides are any compound or substance whose purpose is to kill microbes (e.g. bacteria or viruses). In the context of sexually transmitted infections, microbicides are compounds that can be applied inside the vagina or rectum to protect against sexually transmitted infections including HIV. They can be formulated as gels, creams, films, or suppositories. Not all microbicides have spermicidal activity (a contraceptive effect). An effective microbicide against HIV is not yet available.

[2] *Trichomonas vaginalis* (*T. vaginalis*) is a sexually transmitted infection (STI) and the most common pathogenic protozoan infection of women in industrialized countries.

The study participants were asked to apply the gel or a placebo vaginally at least three times a week and before intercourse for approximately 1 year. Once enrolled in the trial, all women had monthly examinations at the clinic to check for signs of irritation and test for STIs. At these visits the women received safe-sex counselling, free condoms, and counselling to ensure that they understood the trial requirements and objectives. If a woman was found to have a treatable STI she received treatment; every 3 months, the women were tested for HIV and asked a series of questions about product acceptability. If she was found to have HIV or another disease, clinic staff referred her to health and support services (secondary or tertiary hospitals or social workers) available in the local area and encouraged the woman to take her partner with her. Counselling before and after the test was provided in connection with the HIV testing, and women had the option whether to receive their test results or not. Women who were diagnosed as HIV-positive could choose to continue to participate in the trial so that leaving the trial would not signal their HIV serostatus. All participants received modest monetary compensation for time and transport for each visit, as well as refreshments.

At a pre-study meeting, a group of women from the community health committee registered their disagreement with the researchers' decision not to obtain informed consent from the partners of women in the trial. They believe that this action might place women at risk for sexual and physical abuse if their partner discovered their use of the product without their approval. The co-investigators from the host country, who were also present at the meeting, argue that if men were informed about the microbicide, they would not allow their partners to take part in the study. The need for male consent would also negate one purpose of the study, which was to test a female-controlled method.

Questions

1 Should investigators seek informed consent from the women's partners? Should it be required?

2 If a woman becomes HIV-positive during the trial, should her regular partner be informed? What if she has more than one partner? What if she develops an STI other than HIV?

3 If the community health committee does not agree with the decisions being made by the investigators, what can they do to make their voices heard?

4 At the time that this study was planned, anti-retroviral treatment for HIV positive patients who required treatment was not available through the country's health system. HIV surveillance was however routinely carried out without offering back the test results. In the context of this research study, was it ethical to withhold the test results from research participants even if they had consented not to receive them?

Case 26

A study to determine the value of postoperative radiotherapy

Over an 11-year period, a well-respected cancer hospital in East Asia studied a much debated issue: whether the survival of patients with oesophageal cancer is improved by radiotherapy after resection (surgical removal of the cancer cells). The study did not receive an ethics review before it was started because at the time few research institutions in the country had research ethics committees.

Patients at the hospital who underwent radical resection during this period were randomly assigned into two groups: those who only had surgery and those who also received radiotherapy (treatment with radiation to kill any remaining cancer cells), beginning 3-4 weeks after their surgery. Clinicians told patients in the radiotherapy group that they were being given "innovative therapy". The clinicians provided complete descriptions of the probable risks and benefits of the treatment, after which patients had the opportunity to accept or refuse it.

None of the patients were told that they were participants in an experiment. The investigators believed that the population under study had such a strong, culturally rooted distrust of medical science that even simply using the term "research" would trigger a refusal by most patients to participate. The investigators reasoned that since the patients received all the information relevant to whichever intervention they were being offered and were free to accept or refuse that treatment, their oral approval was sufficient to keep the study in compliance with prevailing guidelines for informed consent.

The researchers submitted their results, which lent substantial support for postoperative radiotherapy in the treatment of oesophageal carcinoma, to a well-respected medical journal in the North America. After some deliberation, the journal's editor decided to print the paper but invited an editorial from a North American physician and ethicist who criticized the lack of informed consent and ethical review, adding that violations of human rights were frequent in the country where the study was done. The authors were not shown the editorial nor invited to reply.

Questions

1. Do you agree with the investigators' ethical justification of their decision not to tell patients that they were in an experiment? Why or why not?

2. What harm, if any, did the patients experience because they were not informed that they were participants in a study?

3. Though now widely introduced, formal mechanisms for informed consent and prior ethical review were not standard in the country when the study was done. Is it appropriate to use today's ethical standards to judge a study that began years ago?

4. Should the journal have printed a study that reviewers found unethical? When, if ever, is the scientific value of a study significant enough to justify publication despite ethical violations?

5. Should the authors have been given the opportunity to reply to the editorial?

6. Did the journal editor adopt an ethical approach by publishing an editorial against a published study without informing the investigators?

Case 27

Micronutrient supplementation for pregnant women

Maternal vitamin A deficiency is a major public health problem in South Asia. Premature births and small size for gestational age, both of which are leading risk factors for stillbirths and for neonatal and early childhood death, have been linked to insufficient levels of vitamin A in mothers with low socioeconomic status. A large field trial in Asia has reported a 30% reduction in the mortality rates of preschool children who were given vitamin A supplements. However, whether supplementation to a mother will have a positive effect on her health status and/or that of her infant is unknown.

To address this lack of knowledge, a large randomized double-blind placebo-controlled community based trial is undertaken in a South Asian country with both high levels of poverty and illiteracy and known vitamin A deficiency in infants and women. The purpose of this study is to determine whether a low-dose supplement of vitamin A, or a dose of beta-carotene,[1] given weekly to women of reproductive age will reduce deaths and illness related to pregnancy, and improve the growth and survival of young infants. All married women of reproductive age who live in a randomly selected sample of 270 villages are eligible to participate. Although vitamin A is regarded as a potential teratogen[2] when taken in unusually high doses every day, no known risks have been associated with either the weekly dose of vitamin A or beta-carotene used in this study. The study is given the support of the country's ministry of health, which wants to show that the endemically high prenatal and infant mortality rates are being actively addressed.

Before the start of the study, the investigators hold meetings with the district health officials of the 270 study villages to explain the study in detail. They emphasize that women in a third of the villages will receive a placebo pill with no active ingredient. The district heath officials give permission to start the research. The study is announced in all the villages by a public 'crier' as a ministry of health initiative to decrease newborn mortality and improve their health. Villagers are informed that the community health workers hired for this study in each village will visit them every week and that they should provide these workers with their support. A total of 45 000 women enrol in the study.

Community health workers distribute the test intervention to the women's homes. If women become pregnant, the community health workers take an informed consent from the pregnant woman to allow the pregnancy, mother, and infant to be monitored by the community health workers as part of the research. The women who have signed consent forms are to be interviewed twice during pregnancy and at 3 and 6 months after the delivery of the baby. Women in 27 (10%) of the villages are also invited to have more detailed clinical examinations to assess them for malaria, anaemia, parasitic infections, anthropometry,[3] and diet. The babies of these women are weighed and measured within 10 days of birth. Babies also provide blood samples at 3 months of age, and have detailed measurements of their growth taken at 6 months of age.

Approximately 3 months into the trial, some women complain to the village leaders that they do not wish to take the supplements every week because the drug is a western medicine. The women also tell leaders that they have heard rumours that the supplements do not have any real medicinal effects. They want the village leaders to take up the issue with the rest of the village and stop the trial from taking place.

---

[1] Beta-carotene: an antioxidant found in many vegetables which is partly converted to vitamin A by the liver. Scientists believe that beta-carotene as found in fresh fruit and vegetables has properties that can contribute to reducing cancer and heart disease.

[2] A teratogen is any medication, chemical, infectious disease, or environmental agent that might interfere with the normal development of a fetus and result in the loss of a pregnancy, a birth defect, or a pregnancy complication

[3] Anthropometry is the study of the measurement of the human body in terms of the dimensions of bone, muscle, and adipose (fat) tissue.

Questions

1. Randomization of communities, as opposed to individuals, in a study design can pose technical issues. Does it also pose any ethical issues?

2. Was the consent process adequate? What issues would you have flagged either for more information or for changes if you were a member of a REC asked to review this study?

3. Is it mandatory that participants understand the meaning of randomization?

4. How could the investigators have avoided this situation?

Case 28

Breastfeeding and mother-to-child HIV transmission

> This case is based on research that took place in the 1990s and is not based on recent knowledge. It is included here because the ethical questions remain valid.[1]

A research group based at a medical research institute in a central African country is studying the risk for HIV infection in children who are breastfed by HIV-infected mothers. Should breastfeeding by a HIV-positive mother prove to significantly increase the risk of infection in her infant, existing ministry of health recommendation that mothers should breastfeed regardless of their HIV status would have to change. Findings from a previous study suggested that breastfeeding might be associated with an increase in HIV transmission. However, that study had some design flaws so the investigators at the medical research institute believe that the study needs to be repeated.

The research is being undertaken at the city's general hospital over a 1-year period. With the belief that pregnant women and their partners should jointly make the decision to participate in the study, the researchers seek informed consent from both partners. The consent forms are clear, seemingly comprehensive, and include a clause stating that the participants can opt out of the trial at any time without compromising the health care at the clinic for either mother or child. The researchers offer no inducements to encourage participants to join the study although they are very aware both that antiretroviral drugs are not readily available to most of those who need them in the country and that there is no preventive mother-to-child-transmission programme in the hospital.

At the third trimester prenatal visit for an in-hospital delivery, every participant has blood drawn to determine their HIV status. Before delivery, the women learn of their HIV status. Those who are found to be seropositive receive counselling and are advised not to breastfeed their infants. The counsellors assure them that all the infant formula they need will be provided to them free of charge. Nevertheless, some of the women choose to breastfeed, thereby providing two non-randomly selected groups: the HIV-positive women who choose not to breastfeed are the study group and the HIV-positive women who choose to breastfeed comprise the control group. The HIV status of every child, whether they receive breast milk or infant formula, is assessed at birth and every 6 months up to 18 months; the mother's status is reassessed at 18 months. All children in the study are seen at least every 2 weeks in a special clinic where drugs for common childhood illnesses, as well as for HIV-associated opportunistic infections, are available free of charge.

One of the women seen in the prenatal clinic at week 24 of pregnancy, who had tested positive for HIV, is a healthy 32-year-old married woman with two healthy children (2 and 5 years of age). Her medical history shows that she received a blood transfusion after a postpartum haemorrhage during her last delivery. According to protocol, she is informed of the general benefits of breastfeeding and the countervailing risks of HIV transmission. Her physician advises her to consider alternative options for infant feeding. A week before her expected date of delivery, after several difficult discussions with a health care worker and her husband, she decides that she will breastfeed her child and will continue to participate in the study. Her husband strongly objects and decides to approach the investigator to try to change his wife's decision. He states that he has equal rights to decide whether the child will be breastfed or not and given his understanding that breastfeeding will probably be a danger to his child, he will seek an order from the court to prevent his wife from breastfeeding. He wants his family to remain in the study as it is the only way that they will have access to sufficient quantities of infant formula as an alternative to breast milk.

---

[1] WHO recommends (2006) that HIV-infected women should use exclusive breastfeeding for the first 6 months of a child's life unless replacement feeding is acceptable, feasible, affordable, sustainable, and safe for them and their infants. If those criteria are met, avoidance of all breastfeeding by HIV-infected women is recommended. WHO HIV and Infant Feeding Technical Consultation. Consensus Statement. Geneva, Switzerland: Inter-agency Task Team (IATT) on Prevention of HIV Infections in Pregnant Women, Mothers and their Infants, 2006.

Questions

1. Since only the woman's HIV status is relevant to the risk being studied (transmission of HIV through breastfeeding), is it appropriate to seek informed consent from both the woman and her partner? What if the woman does not wish to reveal her HIV status to her partner?

2. What role should the husband in this case have in the decision about whether or not to breastfeed, given that it could seriously affect the health of his child?

3. Does the provision of free clinic visits every 2 weeks and free medication constitute a form of undue inducement to participate?

4. Given that a previous (albeit flawed) study has already shown a risk of HIV-transmission through breastfeeding, is it appropriate to do this study?

5. Comment on the risk-benefit ratio of this study for participants. Do you see any way to improve the ratio?

6. What is the role of the investigator in this situation? Could the investigator have avoided the situation in which both partners wish to stay in the study but exercise opposite options?

Case 29

Humanized mice

Like malaria, dengue fever is a potentially fatal, mosquito-borne viral disease. Although dengue, with its severe, flu-like symptoms, rarely causes death, dengue haemorrhagic fever, a potentially lethal complication, has become a leading cause of admission to hospital and death among children in several tropical and subtropical countries. Vaccine development for dengue has been difficult because this disease can be caused by one of four related viruses and unless a vaccine can protect against all four, the vaccine could possibly increase the risk of the more serious variant, dengue haemorrhagic fever.

A group of researchers from a South American university want to evaluate the possibility of developing a vaccine for dengue. To improve understanding of the interaction between dengue or dengue haemorrhagic fever, and the immune system, they first develop an animal model of the disease that they plan to test in mice. The mice intended for use in the study are immunodeficient, and human umbilical-cord blood will be used to reconstitute their immune systems. Approximately 100 near-partum women are recruited to take part in the study, in which they need to donate small amounts of umbilical-cord blood. The forms for obtaining informed consent forms state that the "cord blood sample will be sent to a research lab where it will be tested for how well certain blood cells react to foreign substances". Umbilical-cord blood is sent without identification to the researchers, who then inject the samples into the mice. Although the title on the consent form indicated that the samples would be used in studies involving small animal models and the women were welcome to ask any further questions about the study, the consent form did not emphasize that the cord blood would be injected into mice and used to reconstitute their immune systems.

The study was approved by the local research ethics committee. After a year had passed, one woman who donated umbilical-cord blood read an article about "humanized mice" and recalled that she had agreed to participate in a similar study. She complained to her obstetrician and to the administrative coordinator of the committee, stating that she felt cheated by the study because she was not informed by the researchers that her cells would be injected into a mouse.

Citing the clause in the informed consent form that she could end her participation in the research at any time, she insisted on having all her samples retraced and withdrawn from the study immediately.

Questions

1 Was the woman in this study properly informed about the research for which she donated her blood?

2 Since the samples had already been anonymized and injected into the mice, were her requests reasonable?

3 Is there more appropriate information that could have been provided to the women?

Case 30

Donations for stem-cell research

In country X, the government allows the use of human embryos up to 14-days-old for stem-cell research. Researchers often acquire embryos through cooperation with clinical institutes that provide assisted-reproduction services. Embryos are usually collected before a specific research study. The doctor responsible for the assisted-reproduction technology most commonly obtains informed consent from patients to donate "spare" embryos.

In acquiring informed consent, the clinician first talks with the patients to provide basic information about the techniques of assisted reproduction, including the nature of the procedure, the possible risks and benefits, and the legal status of the children produced by this method. The consent form for embryo donation and that for the use of assisted-reproduction technology are merged for efficiency, and because researchers feel that patients' anxiety is reduced by having to sign only one form instead of two.

When reviewing the section of the form that deals with "disposal of surplus embryos", the doctor informs the patients of their options in this matter: freezing or preservation of any embryos that are not implanted, destroying stored embryos after successful reproduction efforts, or provision of embryos for use in stem-cell investigations. The doctor further describes the possible stem-cell procedures and the purposes of such work. The patients are assured that their embryos will not be used for reproductive cloning, although they might be used to advance human welfare if such a study were approved by a research ethics committee. Because of perceived patient sensitivities, specific words such as donation, research, and informed consent are not used in the form or the doctor's explanation.

Questions

1. Can words such as "research" be eliminated from the informed consent form, even if the patients are offered a complete explanation of what procedures might be used for stem-cell investigation?

2. Can one consent form be used to cover the assisted-reproduction procedure and the use of the extra embryos for investigations not connected with the reproductive goal?

3. Can informed consent for the use of biological specimens be obtained for studies that have yet to be defined, and what is the best format for doing so?

Adapted from a case study provided by Misheng F, Lin Z. and included with permission.

Case 31

Researching health care practices and needs in an elderly population

In recent decades, the nomadic populations of the northern Sahara have adopted a more sedentary lifestyle, settling in cities and villages that were once only temporary stopovers. Officials in one regional health district noticed that many elderly members of one of these formerly nomadic communities were admitted to hospital for conditions that were largely preventable or that could have been addressed more appropriately, and at less cost, in outpatient clinics if they had been seen by medical staff earlier. In order to understand how to meet the health care needs of this group of elderly people, and possibly to reduce costs, the regional health district agreed to enter into a research partnership with a European university.

The aim was to use surveys to investigate traditional and existing health care practices, health-related beliefs, and the health needs of the district's elderly nomadic population. Researchers would have access to hospital records. Before beginning the research, the researchers would obtain approval from local authorities and the ethics committees at relevant hospitals.

The study focused on people in the community who were at least 60 years old, virtually all of whom lived with the family of an adult son (the recognized "head of the household"). Aware of the importance of involving the head of the household in any decisions, the researchers began by explaining the study and its purpose to the adult son before asking permission to approach one of their elderly parents about participating in the study. After obtaining consent from each participant in the local language, the interview was conducted in a separate room. To ensure privacy and confidentiality, no family members were in the room with the researcher and participant. The interviews lasted between 60 and 90 minutes.

Midway through one of the interviews with an eighty-year old man, the investigators noticed that the participant had started to tremble and sweat, and had become incoherent. The researcher called the participant's son who reacted angrily, and accused the investigators of being insensitive and callous. He shouted that the researcher had intentionally made his father sick in order to force him into the hospital where he would be over-medicated, instead of being cared for by his family in the traditional manner. He demanded that the researcher leave immediately.

Questions

1. How could this situation have been avoided? Is this situation more specific to elderly people? What are the specific ethical considerations while doing research on the elderly?

2. Was the consent process sufficient to take into consideration the special needs of older people – e.g. cognitive impairment or an underlying medical condition? What ethical framework could be adopted to take this into consideration?

3. Should the ethics committees have reviewed the questions of the survey? What advice could the REC have given the investigators?

Adapted from a case study provided by Dr Astrid Stuckelberger, Department of Social and Community Health at the Faculty of Medicine, University of Geneva, Switzerland.

Chapter V

Standard of Care

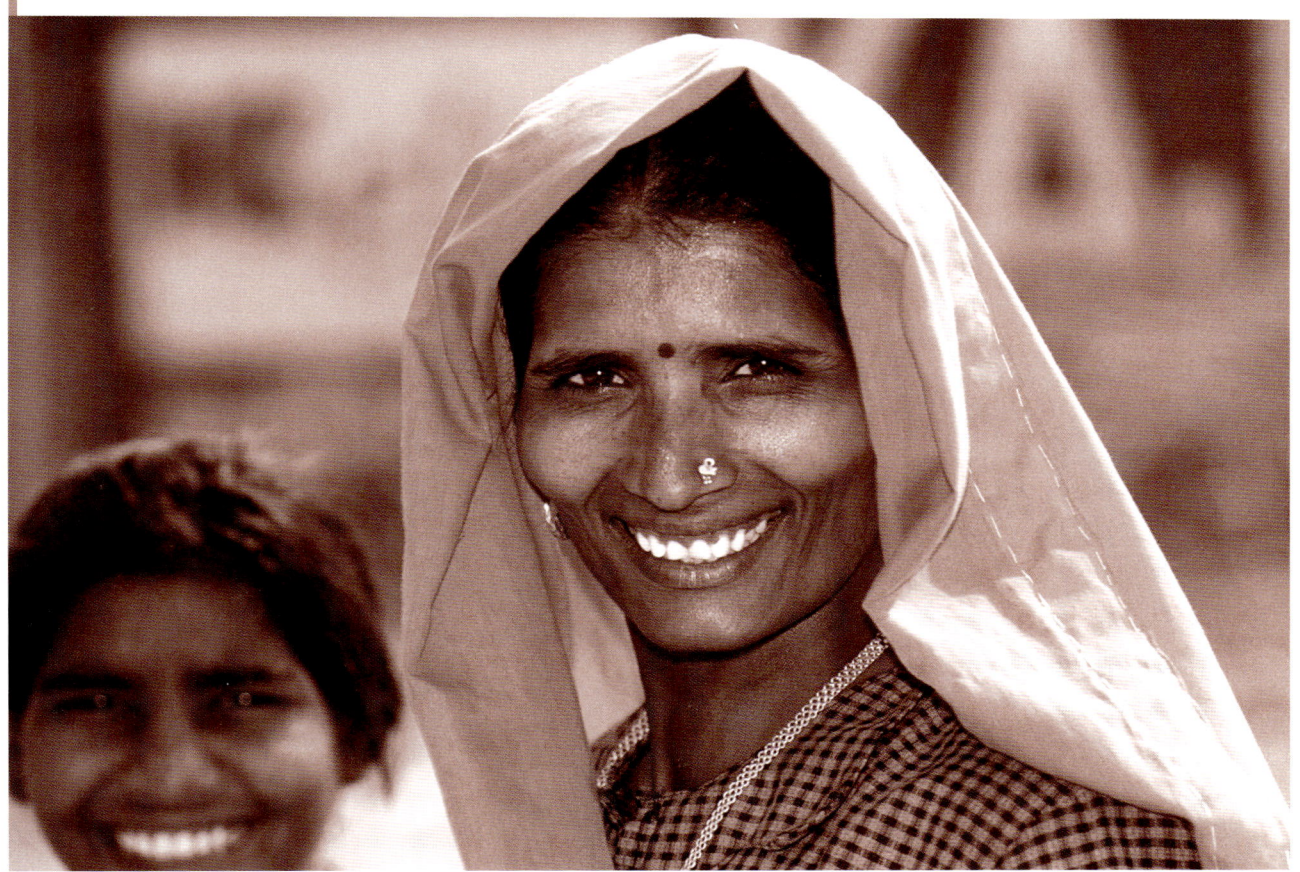

© WHO/Pierre Virot

Introduction: Chapter V

Whose standard?

Some of the most contentious ethical issues in international health research arise in research studies that use a randomized controlled trial (RCT) design to test new methods and treatments. This is especially true in the context of research that is undertaken in developing countries in which people are particularly vulnerable to exploitation. In chapter II, some of these issues, including the use of placebo, were discussed in relation to the study design. This chapter will focus specifically on the standard of care that should be provided to the control group in a randomized controlled trial. A range of viewpoints from a so-called 'global single standard' to a more permissive contextual perspective will be presented. Chapter VI, in turn, will discuss a broader range of ethical issues concerning the care and treatment researchers and other stakeholders in the research process owe to research participants and their communities.

Interpreting the Declaration of Helsinki, Article 32[1]

According to Article 32 of the 2008 edition of the World Medical Association's *Declaration of Helsinki*, which is probably the most influential statement of research ethics principles,

> The benefits, risks, burdens and effectiveness of a new method should be tested against those of the best proven current method, except in the following circumstances:
>
> - the use of placebo, or no treatment, is acceptable in studies where no proven current method exists; or
>
> - where for compelling and scientifically sound methodological reasons the use of placebo is necessary to determine the efficacy or safety of a method and the patients who receive placebo or no treatment will not be subject to any additional risk of serious or irreversible harm.

The *Declaration* makes no reference to local conditions or resource constraints, and can be seen to imply that, irrespective of where experiments are undertaken, the drug or intervention to be tested should be compared with "the best" medical intervention available anywhere in the world at this time. However, as can be seen in Article 32, the *Declaration* contains a limiting clarification: this requirement may be relaxed "[w]here for compelling and scientifically sound methodological reasons the use of placebo is necessary to determine the efficacy or safety of a method and the patients who receive placebo or no treatment will not be subject to any additional risk of serious or irreversible harm." Thus, whenever a means of preventing, diagnosing or treating a condition exists, researchers must provide it to the control group unless there are compelling and persuasive scientific grounds for using a placebo

If one takes this view, then, as many commentators have noted, application of the dictum "should implies can" would mean one of two things. It could be argued that if "the best" care cannot possibly be provided at a particular test site, its provision cannot be morally obligatory. Conversely, Article 32 could be interpreted as forbidding the research project if the highest standard of care could not be provided at the proposed site.

---

[1] Article 29 in previous editions of the DoH, has become Article 32 in the most recent (2008) edition. The wording has changed slightly but the substance remains unchanged.

World Medical Association. Declaration of Helsinki: Ethical Principles for Medical Research Involving Human Subjects. Helsinki, Finland: World Medical Association, 1964. Most recent revised and updated version 2008. http://www.wma.net/e/ethicsunit/helsinki.htm (accessed 5 June 2009)

A different way of interpreting Article 32 would be that a new intervention should be compared against those of the best proven current method available to most patients in the country or at the research site rather than the best world standard of care. In the following paragraphs, the positives and negatives of these interpretations of Article 32 will be discussed.

A single global standard

The 'single-standard' position opposes any double standards that would allow researchers working in a developing country, but who come from a developed country with a high standard of care, to provide research participants with care at the prevailing local standards. A single world standard, in this view, provides moral consistency and is required of anyone who values every life equally, irrespective of the wealth or geographic location of the participant. The single-standard view, proponents argue, is also consistent with the *Declaration of Helsinki*, which gives higher priority to the well-being of research participants than to obtaining scientific information.

The single-standard position does not require the experimental treatment to be the best available, but only that it be tested against the best (i.e. what is provided to the control group in the trial). Therefore, the single-standard view would allow trials of less expensive treatments, even if they are prospectively recognized as inferior to the best treatments available somewhere in the world, on the proviso that participants in the control group of the study receive the best possible care. This position has at least two unfortunate consequences.

First, placebo-controlled trials of low-cost alternatives would be ruled out when an effective remedy is available elsewhere, even if the latter treatment could not be adopted in the country where the trial is held for reasons of expense, absence of necessary infrastructure, or lack of trained personnel. Exclusion of a placebo-controlled trial in such circumstances would mean that a poor country would be precluded from establishing which low-cost alternatives offer valuable medical benefits, even if they were not as beneficial as the (unattainable) existing therapy. Such a low-cost alternative might prove to be beneficial (and could then be accepted for licensing and use) were tested in a placebo-controlled RCT and shown to be better than a placebo, even if it would have failed if tested against the highest global standard of care in an equivalency or superiority trial.

Second, the single-standard interpretation of Article 32 is open to further challenge, since trials of substantially inferior treatments, even costly ones, seem to be allowed as long as participants in the control group receive the best available treatment. That type of trial would clearly contravene the ethical principle embodied in Article 32, (that all participants in research should have access to the best medical interventions currently available in the world), which raises questions about the defence of the single-standard view. More important, testing against the best global treatment when it is not otherwise available locally would mean that researchers would be making the treatment available to participants in the trial, which might create an inducement for impoverished people to enrol in the trial. Further inequities could be exacerbated within such a population, since the treatments available through research would be far better than those available through the health system (which might actually be no treatment).

Highest sustainable standard

Most of the criticism of the single-standard view has focused on the impracticality of the provision of world-class health care in resource-poor settings. However, the second interpretation of the *Declaration of Helsinki* can be taken to mean the highest standard of care available where the research will be conducted or that can be sustained there. This interpretation provides investigators in resource-poor settings with the moral basis to test low-cost alternatives against a placebo since the prevalent standard in the country might be no treatment, even if an effective treatment of the disease did exist elsewhere in the world. For impoverished populations, the availability of high-cost drugs or other interventions is immaterial to health problems, whereas an alternative that carries a low or very low cost, might make the difference between good health and death or disability, even if the treatment is medically inferior to the best available elsewhere. Others argue that this understanding would allow several standards, since standards and health care vary substantially among developing countries. What one country regards as sustainable, therefore, might be viewed by another as unaffordable. Moreover, some countries that offer very little to most of their citizens manage to sustain a high level of care in one or more hospitals and clinics that serve the economic and political elite. 'Sustainability' might turn out to be less a *fact* and more a political *decision*.

Prevailing local standard

The least demanding interpretation would require only that the standard of care in an experiment be no lower than that which prevails for the participants' population at the test site rather than nationally. This requirement would be enough to ensure that participants would receive care that is at least as good as what they would have received had they not been enrolled in the research study. As long as a research study did not worsen the health of participants compared with their prospects outside the study, it could be allowed to go ahead. Under this interpretation, investigators would also be permitted to use opportunities for natural experiments with participants who would not otherwise be available for study, such as pharmacologically naïve patients who had never received vaccines or drugs that are commonly available to most of the population, even in developing countries.

The chief objection to this standard, which at one time was proposed (but rejected) as a replacement for Article 29 (now Article 32) of the *Declaration of Helsinki*, is that it allows researchers to offer no more than whatever happens to be the status quo at the test site, even if that standard is no care. Populations that do not receive adequate health care services, or those that most people would agree deserve much better care than they have been receiving, would still continue to be under-served in the research study. In effect, researchers and sponsors would be perpetuating, even exploiting, the social injustices that exist at the test site. Indeed, use of this standard could be viewed as an incentive to sponsors to seek test sites in which injustices are greatest, since they would have to provide little or nothing to participants. Conducting research in such settings could prove to be very cost-effective for research sponsors, both because less care has to be provided to study participants and because they might be less demanding and less likely to be well protected by institutions that would advocate for their welfare.

The standard of care for treatment of incidental conditions

What standard of care should be provided for treatment of conditions other than the one that is the object of research? For example, in a study designed to establish the blood levels of commonly used anti-tuberculosis drugs, what standard of care should be provided to patients who are found to have other incidental diseases? Or, what standard of care should be provided to research participants who are included in a study to measure the effect of changing behaviour on the progression of their disease? What standard of care should be provided to those participants if other incidental diseases be detected during the study? In these situations, should participants receive the best current treatment during their involvement, even though that is not the national standard? If that were offered, would the investigators not create further inequities in a country that already has limited resources and is likely to have many existing inequities? If participants are excluded from a trial because the investigators tested for and diagnosed a disease or disorder that meets criterion for exclusion from the study, what treatment, if any, would the investigators be obliged to provide and at what standard of care? For how long should such treatment be provided if the condition uncovered is chronic or not quickly cured? If the disease detected is hereditary, does any such duty of care extend to other relatives? Finally, why should the investigators have to uphold a standard of care that the countries themselves cannot uphold, especially since they would not otherwise have a responsibility to treat diseases incidental to the study?

Many investigators and ethicists have argued that the principles of beneficence and justice require that investigators have some responsibility for the physical, social, and mental well-being of participants in their research, and therefore that in these and other similar situations they should take some responsibility for the research participants – or even people who were willing to participate but who were excluded because of other diseases or disorders. Although many of these issues could be regarded as ancillary-care issues (i.e. not directly related to research; see chapter VI for further discussion), others have argued that research does not occur in a vacuum, and that researchers and sponsors from resource-rich nations have a broader role, especially when they seek to carry out research in resource-poor settings. Researchers and sponsors can discharge their responsibility to contribute to improving the health care of the population by creative collaborations with various stakeholders before the start of any study, with the aim of making a lasting contribution to the goal of raising the standard of care in the host country.

Suggested readings

Killen J, et al. Ethics of Clinical Research in the Developing World. *Nature Reviews*, 2002, 2: 210-215.

"Many commentators believe that all clinical trial participants must receive a level of care equivalent to the world's best. Using HIV/AIDS research as an example, [the authors] show how this 'Uniform Care Requirement' can undermine biomedical research aimed at improving global health, and then [they] point towards a more rational and balanced approach to ethical assessment."

http://dx.doi.org/10.1038/nri745
(accessed 25 August 2008)

Kottow MH. Who Is My Brother's Keeper? *Journal of Medical Ethics*, 2002, 28:24-27.

"Recent years have witnessed frequent reports of less stringent ethical standards being applied to both clinical and research medical practices initiated by developed countries in poorer nations. Still more unsettling, a number of articles have endorsed the policy of employing ethical norms in these host countries, which would be unacceptable to both the legislations and the moral standards of the sponsor nations". The author expresses his concern for the support and approval that is being accorded by bioethicists to the application of differential standards.

http://jme.bmj.com/cgi/content/full/28/1/24
(accessed 9 May 2008)

Wolinsky H. The Battle of Helsinki: Two Troublesome Paragraphs in the Declaration of Helsinki are Causing a Furor over Medical Research Ethics. *European Molecular Biology Organization*, 2006 7(7):670-672.

"Later this year, the US Food and Drug Administration plans to rewrite its regulations to eliminate any reference to the Declaration of Helsinki (DoH), a document from the World Medical Association […] that many consider to be the hallmark of medical ethics. This decision, triggered by the 2000 update to the DoH, is the latest move in an increasingly heated debate over medical research ethics. The FDA is reacting in particular to the addition of two controversial paragraphs, which, if adopted in their own regulations, would limit the use of placebos in drug trials and increase the responsibilities of trial sponsors towards research participants." This article presents the arguments and politics concerning the changes to the DoH.

http://dx.doi.org/10.1038/sj.embor.7400743
(accessed 25 August 2008)

Case 32

Testing a new HIV vaccine

> This case is based on research conducted in the 1990s when antiretroviral drugs were not generally available in most developing countries and the standard of care described here was the prevailing standard.

In 1998, Vidavax, a pharmaceutical company based in northern Europe, developed an HIV vaccine that appeared promising. Animal studies were very successful, and phase I and II trials demonstrated that the vaccine was remarkably safe and produced significant antibody levels in nearly all volunteers. The company then wanted to begin phase III trials in a South-East Asian country where previous surveillance had identified a cohort of intravenous drug users who had a high rate of seroconversion.

The government of the South-East Asian country expressed interest in having the study done in their jurisdiction and began negotiations with Vidavax. The vaccine, which was specifically directed against the strain of HIV that predominates in that country's population of intravenous drug users, would be provided free by the pharmaceutical company. Vidavax would also cover the cost of the study, which would be undertaken by the vaccine institute in the South-East Asian country. In addition to the study costs, the pharmaceutical company would provide all of the necessary laboratory equipment, ten computers for the institute, and two vehicles for visits to the study sites. The company further agreed that if the vaccine proved effective it would be given free of charge to intravenous drug users in the city and at cost to the country for 5 years.

This was to be a randomized double-blind prospective study, with one group receiving the test vaccine and the other receiving a placebo. All potential participants were to be tested for HIV before being enrolled in the study. If they tested positive for the virus, they would be referred to one of the municipal hospitals. The company and the vaccine institute also agreed that anyone who contracted HIV during the study would likewise be referred to one of the municipal hospitals and treated according to the standards established by the ministry of health. These standards stipulated treatment for all infections, although participants were not given antiretroviral drugs, including zidovudine (AZT) or protease inhibitors. Should the government make any changes to the recommended standard of treatment during the study, all seroconvertors would be switched to the new therapy. The municipality would provide its treatment for the lifetime of the seroconverted participants.

The informed consent process would have two stages. In the first stage, researchers would brief potential participants about the study and explain both the experimental nature of the vaccine and the treatment policy. The individuals would return to the institute 2 days after the initial briefing for brief oral and written exams to certify their full understanding of the study and their rights. Only participants whose tests showed that they had a strong understanding of the study and their rights would be enrolled. Individuals were informed that they could drop out at any time without fear of prejudice.

The investigators submitted the study proposal to the institute's research ethics committee and to a firm that conducts ethical reviews of proposals involving human subject research for private companies. The protocol was also reviewed informally and commented on by an international organization, at the request of the ministry of health's technical subcommittee on HIV vaccines. The subcommittee approved the protocol and forwarded it to the health ministry's research ethics committee. All review committees approved the study.

After the study commenced, an article condemning the trial appeared in an AIDS activist group's publication. The group objected to the fact that the study would not provide state-of-the-art care for seroconverting individuals. They argued that the only reason to do the study in South-East Asia was because the health ministry's treatment guidelines did not require antiretroviral therapy. The article contended that in a developed country, neither a government nor the research ethics committee of a university would approve the study proposal. Vidavax countered that the use of state-of-the-art treatment would in itself be unethical because the treatment regimen would not be sustainable in the study country and only one small group would have access to antiretroviral drugs. The country did not want to offer therapy to only one small group, and at the time the country was unwilling to offer treatment to the entire population. Finally, the researchers argued that provision of state-of-the-art care that the participants would not otherwise have access to would constitute unfair inducement to participate in the study.

Questions

1. Is this study ethical? Discuss.

2. Would it be ethical to offer state-of-the-art care to participants who were seroconvertors even if the care was not generally available in the country?

3. Is there a compromise position that might be acceptable to both parties?

4. Should any other services be provided to the population of intravenous drug users?

5. Is it appropriate for the company to offer computers, vehicles, and lab equipment to the vaccine institute?

6. If the developer of the vaccine were a South-East Asian company that wished to do the study in its own country, would the use of "best available or standard local therapy" for seroconvertors be viewed differently? What are the implications if the standards are different? What are the implications if the standards are the same?

Case 33

Short-course antiretroviral therapy in pregnant women

Viraret is an antiretroviral drug that is manufactured in Europe. A study in a southern African country was undertaken to test the efficacy of the drug for prevention of vertical transmission of HIV when given in an innovative, short-course (one dose) regimen to pregnant women who were HIV-positive. The study, which was conducted under the auspices of a prestigious European institute concerned with prevention of transmissible diseases, aimed to offer a rough picture of efficacy, not to serve as a stand-alone study for drug-licensing purposes. However, data for efficacy from the trial were so compelling that WHO stated that further trials would be unethical and endorsed the use of Viravet as a single-dose therapy for pregnant women with AIDS to prevent mother-to-child transmission of the disease.

The government of an east African country, through its drug regulatory authority, then took steps to license Viraret for use. However, a re-examination of the original data from the European institute showed defects in the study's compliance with Good Clinical Practice.[1] The discovery of these defects meant that the study provided an insufficient basis for the European regulatory authority to license the product for the prevention of vertical transmission of HIV. Citing a requirement that drugs proposed for licensing in the east African country must also be licensed in the country where they are manufactured, the regulatory authority refused to license the product. Nevertheless, WHO reaffirmed its recommendations for Viravet. Subsequently the regulatory authority bowed to international pressure and licensed the drug.

Questions

1. Is the opinion of the European regulatory agency relevant to the decision of the African country's drug regulatory authority?

2. If so, what alternative action could the regulatory authority have taken?

3. What was the role of WHO in this situation? Was it appropriate?

4. What actions could have been taken by the partners involved to avoid such a situation?

Adapted from a case study contributed by Dr J Milstien, Center for Vaccine Development, University of Maryland School of Medicine, Baltimore, MD, USA.

---

[1] Good Clinical Practice (GCP) is an international ethical and scientific quality standard for designing, conducting, recording and reporting trials that involve the participation of human subjects. It is termed good clinical practice (although it describes good research practice) to distinguish it from the standards set for good laboratory and good manufacturing practices. WHO has provided guidelines for GCP (Guidelines for good clinical practice (GCP) for trials on pharmaceutical products. WHO Expert Committee on the Use of Essential Drugs. Sixth Report. Geneva, World Health Organization, 1995 (WHO Technical Report Series, No. 850), Annex 3 http://whqlibdoc.who.int/trs/WHO_TRS_850.pdf (accessed 4 June 2009).

The International Conference on Harmonisation of Technical Requirements for Registration of Pharmaceuticals for Human Use (ICH) has also developed GCP guidelines, and the purpose of the ICH GCP Guideline is to provide a unified standard for the European Union (EU), Japan and the United States http://www.ich.org/LOB/media/MEDIA482.pdf (accessed 9 May 2008)

Case 34

Use of quinacrine for non-surgical sterilization

> Although this case is based on research that occurred more than a decade ago, the issues raised by the case remain relevant.[1]

Little access to, and widespread non-compliance with, existing methods of contraception have led to a large unmet need for better options for family planning, especially in developing countries. Surgical sterilization, although safe and effective, is not accessible to all women who want it, especially those in rural or remote areas where trained staff and facilities are generally not available. This lack of accessibility has sparked a worldwide demand for non-surgical sterilization.

The non-surgical, permanent method that has received the most attention – and that has caused the most controversy – is intrauterine application of quinacrine hydrochloride. Although quinacrine has never received regulatory drug approval as a sterilization method for women in any country, proponents of the method claim that it is safe, effective, simple, and inexpensive. They promote quinacrine as a "low cost" (about US$ 1 per dose) procedure that could make sterilization more accessible to women in resource-poor settings, enabling them to avoid unwanted pregnancies and simultaneously decrease the morbidity and mortality associated with unsafe abortion.

Orally administered quinacrine was used for more than 50 years to prevent and treat malaria. Although no longer used for this purpose, it is still given orally to treat several parasitic and inflammatory diseases. Investigation into quinacrine's potential use for female sterilization began in the 1960s in South America, where researchers explored using it as a sclerosing agent[2] to cause scar tissue in the fallopian tubes. This investigation continued in collaboration with a research organization based in the United States of America throughout the 1970s and 1980s. In the late 1970s, the drug was formulated into pellets for insertion through the cervix, either using an apparatus modified from that used to insert an intrauterine device[3] or a similar apparatus. Over the course of several decades, approximately 104 500 women in more than 20 countries (mostly in East and South-East Asia) have been sterilized by this method, but it was never registered for use.

In the 1980s, a North American regulatory agency allowed small-scale clinical trials of quinacrine as a method of sterilization. Investigators affiliated with a North American NGO conducted these trials in women in the United States of America and elsewhere before a hysterectomy. Although some trials continued, the NGO suspended its involvement in 1990, primarily because it was concerned about the potential relationship between quinacrine use and cancer, since a cluster of cancer cases had occurred in quinacrine trials in South America. Independent lab tests in the United States of America suggested that quinacrine causes cells to mutate, providing circumstantial evidence that it might cause cancer.

In the early 1990s, the technique gained widespread attention after the report of a study in South-East Asia involving more than 30 000 cases of quinacrine-pellet insertion for tubal occlusion.[4] Shortly after this report was published, concern about the widespread global use of a drug that was neither fully investigated nor well understood led several highly respected health organizations to review the research on the use of quinacrine for sterilization. All the organizations concluded that, pending further lab research, quinacrine should not be used to sterilize women in any country.

---

[1] This case is based on the same research study as Case 22 but raises a different set of issues and questions.

[2] A substance that causes marked tissue irritation and/or clotting inside a blood vessel, with subsequent local inflammation and tissue destruction.

[3] A small object that is inserted through the cervix and placed in the uterus to prevent pregnancy.

[4] A surgical procedure for permanently terminating a woman's fertility by blocking the fallopian tubes (via tying and cutting, rings, clips or electrocautery), preventing sperm from reaching the ova and causing fertilization.

Increasing public knowledge about the use of quinacrine for sterilization, coupled with scientific confirmation of the mutagenicity of quinacrine, generated notable public outcry in many countries. Women's advocacy groups began to question the ethical legitimacy of quinacrine research. They raised concerns about experimentation on women, particularly women from developing countries, in the absence of adequate preclinical toxicology data. Furthermore, they questioned whether women receiving quinacrine had been advised that the method was experimental and had been given other information and alternatives that were sufficient to ensure informed choice.

These efforts continued until recently, when a backlash largely attributable to a journal article published outside of the scientific press triggered a series of events that effectively stopped the manufacture and global distribution of quinacrine pellets. Specifically, in rapid succession: (1) the sole manufacturer of quinacrine pellets discontinued production; (2) countries that had previously been involved in quinacrine research announced a moratorium on clinical trials related to sterilization; (3) some resource-poor countries criminalized the sale or free distribution of quinacrine pellets for contraceptive use; and (4) in the United States of America, a national regulatory agency issued a warning letter about the drug's safety and ordered distribution of quinacrine pellets to cease and supplies held by specific individuals in that country to be destroyed.

Questions

1. Should a double standard regarding drug safety and efficacy be allowed when it comes to contraceptive risk-benefit ratios because of differences in the ability of developed and developing countries to cope with, and to modify, population growth?

2. Can national and local risk-benefit analyses determine the appropriateness of quinacrine sterilization in a specific setting?

3. Are there situations when such "double standards" may be appropriate and necessary (cf. Case study 18)? Who can make that decision?

Case 35

Investigation of vaginal microbicides

An east African country has a scattered network of community family-planning clinics that provide free access to family-planning methods, maternity-related services, and some diagnosis and care for sexually transmitted infections (STIs); however, patients must pay for any medications, and physicians at these clinics often write prescriptions for drugs that patients cannot afford. The clinics also do not offer Papanicolaou (Pap) smears[1] for cervical cancer, since they do not have the equipment or personnel to perform them.

A group of researchers have received a grant from a foreign health agency to carry out a multi-site, randomized controlled trial at some of the country's family-planning clinics to test the effectiveness of a vaginal microbicide[2] for prevention of HIV transmission in women. Study participants will be routinely tested and treated for viral and bacterial STIs. They will also get annual Pap smears, and appropriate medications for most disorders (including STIs) will be provided free of charge. Women who present with problems unrelated to the study, such as diarrhoea and malaria, will be referred to a clinician on the study team and will receive necessary treatment without charge. The researchers say that the funders have provided support at this level in previous trials, on the basis that research participants are owed the "standard of care" that they would receive in the sponsor's country. The study protocol does not specify whether, and if so how, access to this level of care would be provided after completion of the 3-year trial.

The informational material that will be provided to potential participants explains the possible benefits and harms in detail; before giving informed consent the women must demonstrate, through their answers to a short questionnaire, that they comprehend basic facts about the study. Nonetheless, a member of the research ethics committee has expressed concern that women might not carefully weigh the risks and benefits but instead will join the study simply to get health services not otherwise available to them. This concern about unfair inducement is echoed in reverse in a report from the community advisory board for the family-planning network, which states that women served by the clinics who were not eligible to join similar studies in the past have voiced frustration that this kept them from having access to the same quality of health care services.

Questions

1. How would you define "unfair inducement"? Does the provision of this level of care present an "unfair inducement" to participate in the research?

2. How would you address the concerns of the women who have not been chosen to participate in the study?

3. Given the background level of care, should the study be conducted in this country?

Adapted from the case study titled "Standard of Care: A Case Study. HIV Prevention Trials" provided by Katherine Shapiro

---

[1] A routine screening test used for the detection of early cervical abnormalities, namely precancerous dysplastic changes of the uterine cervix, together with viral, bacterial, and fungal infections of the cervix and vagina. Cervical screening is a relatively simple, low cost and non-invasive method. Regular screening for cervical cancer reduces both the mortality and incidence of cervical carcinoma.

[2] Vaginal microbicides are chemical agents used topically by women within the vagina in order to prevent infection by HIV and potentially by other enveloped viruses and sexually transmitted pathogens. Prototype microbicides are designed to be inserted prior to sexual intercourse and could also be contraceptive, although most current potential microbicides are not.(Weber J, Desai K, Darbyshire J, on behalf of the Microbicides Development Programme (2005) The Development of Vaginal Microbicides for the Prevention of HIV Transmission. PLoS Med 2(5): e142 doi:10.1371/journal.pmed.0020142). The development of vaginal microbicide assumes great significance in the context of the HIV epidemic, because an effective microbicide would be an effective women-controlled method. Condoms, though very effective against the transmission of HIV remain under the control of the male partner.

Chapter VI

Obligations to Participants and Communities

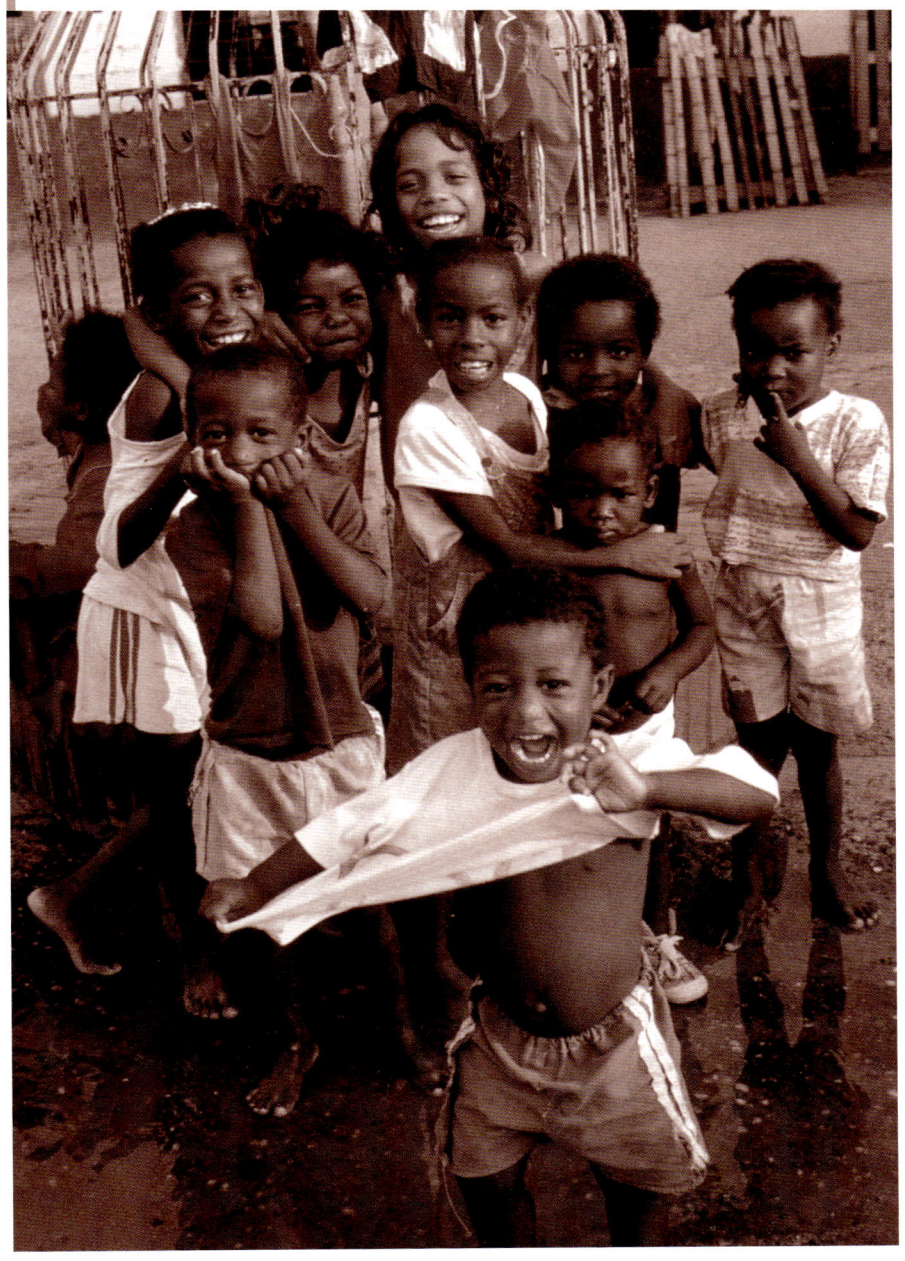

© WHO

Introduction: Chapter VI

How far do researchers' and sponsors' duties extend?

Health research is increasingly understood as a partnership between interested stakeholders – potential and actual volunteers and their communities, funders, sponsors, researchers, and health systems. In order for such a partnership to work well, the expectations and obligations of each stakeholder must be clear from the outset. Anticipation and negotiation of any health-related issues concerning the research can reduce sources of possible conflict and build a positive research relationship.

Although clarity about respective duties and obligations is always important, it takes on an even higher priority for research that is conducted in countries where access to health care and an institutionalized system of delivery are either absent or under-developed. For example, a clinical trial is not part of the health care system, but potential participants might want to enrol because it offers them their only opportunity for care (and perhaps cure). Similarly, researchers might be seen by the population as not only able to provide health care but as obligated to do so, particularly if they are qualified health care personnel such as doctors or nurses and other options for care do not exist. Of course, the opposite situation can also occur, in which participants risk being exploited because they are unaware of their rights, and therefore have very low expectations regarding researchers' and sponsors' obligations to provide care.

Ought stakeholders in the research process do all they can to provide care to participants, and what are their obligations to do so? What do those who instigate and carry out research owe to participants in return for their participation? Do obligations exist to the communities that become research sites, either after consultation and explicit agreement, or by chance? Under what circumstances may research be done in communities which have no existing medical infrastructure (i.e. clinics, dispensaries, hospitals)? What kind of provisions for health care should researchers make before beginning their research?

A range of possible obligations

The question of obligations for prevention and treatment also arise in connection with the so-called "standard of care" debate (see Chapter V). What level of health care should be provided to participants during the course of a study, and in particular should participants in a control group be given a placebo (or in effect, no treatment)? Obligations could relate to the needs of various groups and these are elaborated below:

- The need for care and follow-up for those who are excluded from a study because they have health problems – for example, if high blood sugar is an exclusion criterion for a study to test a new drug against TB, is the researcher conducting the study obligated to provide care to those with high blood sugar, or to ensure that care is available?

- The need for treatment and follow-up for those who must drop out of a trial because they have reached the trial's predefined end-point (for example, altered liver function tests).

- The need for care for participants who are screened for a particular disease in order to develop better and more sensitive diagnostic tests. From the research perspective, the scientist only needs to get initial samples from these participants, and the research findings are unlikely to benefit them directly.

- The need for health care and other types of compensation for participants who are injured during research whether as a direct result of the research or not. Do such obligations differ in countries that have universal health coverage and highly developed social welfare systems as a right of citizenship (rehabilitation services and a programme for lost-wage compensation for example), compared with countries in which no such systems exists?

- The need for continuing care for research participants at the conclusion of a study. Is there an obligation to continue to provide an intervention that the research shows to be effective for a chronic condition to participants who otherwise – because of cost – would not have access to it? If the scientists do not have funding to do so, have they abandoned their patients, in violation of the common prohibition in medical ethics that physicians should not desert their patients partway through treatment? In a randomized controlled trial that identifies one intervention as superior – perhaps the existing "world-class" treatment rather than the treatment that was being tested in the trial – should this intervention be offered at the trial's conclusion to all participants in the study?

- The health needs of participants arising from existing or new medical conditions that are not directly relevant to the research. For example, in one African country, a number of highly trained paediatricians began surveillance for an epidemiological study. In the absence of any other local paediatricians, residents began to bring sick children to the researchers for care. Although the paediatricians had conceived of their mission as one of pure science, they recognized the practical necessity of a compromise and began to offer some patient care. If they had persisted in their initial refusal to provide care without putting their scientific work at risk, would they have been wrong to do so? And how much of the scientific work might justifiably be abandoned – at what cost to future patients' need for the results of the research – to spend time caring for local children?

- The health needs of participants' family members and others in the community where a study is being conducted. For example, in a study that provides supplementary nutrients to infants in a poor village, should the infants' older siblings also be provided with supplements, even though they are not registered participants?

- The need of participants and their communities for information about the results of research and for post-research access to drugs and other products that are proven through the research to be effective.

Guiding ethical principles[1]

If the principles of beneficence (the ethical obligation to maximize benefit and minimize harm) and nonmaleficence (to do no harm) were liberally applied, then researchers and sponsors might be required to respond fully to all of these potential needs and obligations. Is it reasonable, however, to apply these principles so expansively to the scope of the obligations or the range of people to whom they apply? Some would argue that this would make research unaffordable, and that, even if it were affordable for certain sponsors, it would overstep the bounds of research into the realm of health system policy and practice. Others hold that researchers should provide whatever is fairly negotiated among all the stakeholders before the start of the research. In either case, reference to the principles of respect for persons and justice should also be considered in the decision.

[1] See Appendix for a description of each of these guiding principles.

Take, for example, what might seem the easiest case for a duty between researcher and participant – namely when a research participant suffers an injury as a result of his or her participation in a study. In some countries, investigators and sponsors are not obligated to provide any care beyond taking necessary steps to save a participant's life or to prevent grievous harm, provided that when they obtained consent, they had disclosed both the known risks and the absence of any compensation in the case of injury. Under such a regimen, deference to participants' autonomy – their free choice to enrol in research without any promise of compensation for injury – is taken to mitigate the duty to do no harm (nonmaleficence). Yet even here, a participant cannot consent to negligent acts by an investigator, so that an injured participant could still receive compensation through a malpractice suit should the injury have arisen from the investigator's failure to exercise due care under the circumstances.

This very narrow and restrictive conception of obligation and autonomy, relies on the existence of a system of alternative care and an accessible system of justice. In situations with no ready access to a health care system, and where a regulatory system of justice is not to be counted on, obligation, beneficence, autonomy, and justice might require a more sensitive interpretation and application.

Relating obligations to the nature of the relationships

Perceptions of the extent of researchers' obligations to participants, and by extension to other people in their household or community, might depend on how one characterizes the relationships that underlie a research study. An investigator can be seen as having a very limited relationship with the research participants, one that is restricted to their being mutual stakeholders (each in their own special roles) in the research project. So viewed, the relationship would narrowly confine investigators and participants to roles related to the research, and therefore would only carry obligations related to the successful completion of the research project. Thus, for example, no duty to provide care would arise as to ancillary conditions not related to the research.

Alternatively, a researcher may be seen as a care-giving physician or other health care professional in relationship to participants who are also patients with a wide range of medical conditions as well as other problems and needs. For example, research participants often wish to see all members of their families (or communities) fairly treated. This alternative view might be particularly compelling in settings where an investigator is also a participant's treating physician, or where a research project establishes a clinic in a community where health care had not been readily accessible.

Once the relationships between researchers and research participants have been clarified, the implications for research sponsors will need to be addressed. Are sponsors obligated to fund any care that researchers feel they have a professional duty to provide (e.g. for health problems that arise during a project that have no apparent connection to the intervention under study)? Do the financial benefits that the sponsors stand to reap from the research create obligations for them even in circumstances in which investigators do not incur professional duties? How should the obligations of investigators and sponsors regarding needs not directly related to the research be seen in light of the obligations of other local health care professionals and institutions, or of the national government or international governmental and nongovernmental organizations to provide health services?

Looking for solutions, negotiated and principled

In recent years, individual commentators and bioethics commissions alike have ascribed to health researchers an obligation to provide benefits to host communities that go beyond any benefits that may arise from the research itself. Though proposals vary, the specific nature of the benefits seems to matter less than their net value. A sponsor might provide training for health care staff, for example, and leave behind a fully equipped laboratory; or a pharmaceutical company might agree to make any products that a trial shows to be effective available within the host country at cost. These potential benefits can and should be negotiated by the scientists and their sponsors with representatives of the host government, communities, and institutions before a research study begins. Care must be taken, of course, to ensure that the benefits being agreed upon are commensurate both with the value of the research project and with the burdens it imposes on the participants and sites. Benefits should also be designed to reach those most directly involved. Benefits, such as travel and training grants or specialized equipment for local scientists and physicians, might be a means of serving the good of research participants and their communities, or they might be little more than bribes provided to influential elites within the country as a means of getting foreign researchers entry to research sites in communities.

When health research is carried out at sites where many people have no access to the care they need, every contribution to the relief of their health burden can be very valuable, irrespective of its source. The contentious issue is whether investigators who do biomedical research and their sponsors have specific obligations to provide these benefits. If so, how can the extent of these obligations be determined in a non-arbitrary way? Although some scientists and sponsors might have "deep pockets", and individuals in need might turn to them for assistance in the absence of other health services, the result can be that potential sponsors of health research decide that fulfilling such obligations to provide community benefits make that research too expensive to undertake.

RECs will need to decide the extent to which they become involved, either through establishing certain expectations for the level of commitment from researchers and sponsors to improving the circumstances of participants and the community, or through becoming directly involved in negotiations between researchers and sponsors and community representatives. The role a REC plays will depend upon a number of factors, such as the range of authority of that body that appointed the committee, the presence or absence of other groups with the experience and knowledge to play the role of negotiator for the community, and the ease with which the community or its representatives can assemble to negotiate with the researcher and sponsor.

Suggested readings

Andanda PA. Human-Tissue-Related Inventions: Ownership and Intellectual Property Rights in International Collaborative Research in Developing Countries. *Journal of Medical Ethics*, 2008; 34: 3, 171-179.

"There are complex unresolved ethical, legal and social issues related to the use of human tissues obtained in the course of research or diagnostic procedures and retained for further use in research…. It is important for research ethics committees to tread carefully when reviewing research protocols that raise such issues for purposes of ensuring that appropriate benefit sharing agreements, particularly with developing countries, are in place. This paper attempts to analyse the key questions related to ownership and intellectual property rights in commercially viable products derived from human tissue samples."

http://dx.doi.org/10.1136/jme.2006.019612
(accessed 25 August 2008)

Belsky L, Richardson HS. Medical Researchers' Ancillary Clinical Care Responsibilities. *British Medical Journal*, 2004;328:1494-1496.

"Investigation of participants in clinical trials may identify conditions unrelated to the study. Researchers need guidance on whether they have a duty to treat such conditions." Arguing that existing guidelines do not adequately address the ancillary care issues and responsibilities arising during health research, the authors propose an ethical framework that will help delineate researchers' responsibilities.

http://dx.doi.org/10.1136/bmj.328.7454.1494
(accessed 25 August 2008)

MacNeil DS, Fernandez CV. Offering Results to Research Participants. *British Medical Journal*, 2006;332(7535):188.

"Do participants of research trials wish to be offered a summary of the trial results? This practice is being encouraged as a means of demonstrating greater respect for research participants: it recognizes the central role of participants in the completion of research studies and avoids treating them as a means to an end." This editorial recognizes the importance of exercising caution and judgment in the provision of individual research results to participants and supports providing results to those who want them.

http://dx.doi.org/10.1136/bmj.332.7535.188
(accessed 25 August 2008)

Participants in the 2001 Conference on Ethical Aspects of Research in Developing Countries. Ethics: Fair Benefits for Research in Developing Countries. *Science* 2002;298(5601):2133-2134.

"Collaborative, multinational clinical research, especially between developed and developing countries, has been the subject of controversy. Much of this attention has focused on the standard of care used in randomized trials. Much less discussed, but probably more important in terms of its impact on health, is the claim that, in order to avoid exploitation, interventions proven safe and effective through research in developing countries should be made "reasonably available" in those countries."

http://dx.doi.org/10.1126/science.1076899
(accessed 9 May 2008)

Potts M. Thinking About Vaginal Microbicide Testing. *American Journal of Public Health*. 2000;90(2).

"A vaginal microbicide could slow the spread of HIV. To date, volunteers in placebo-controlled trials of candidate microbicides have been counseled to use condoms. This does not reduce the number of volunteers exposed to possible risk, but shifts the allotment of risk from those conducting the trial to those women who may be least able to make autonomous decisions. Alternative ways of meeting the obligation to offer volunteers active benefits are explored." This controversial article challenges accepted practice and generated numerous responses on the issue of condom provision and counseling in microbicide trials.

http://www.ajph.org/cgi/reprint/90/2/188
(accessed 8 April 2009)

Shapiro K, Benatar SR. HIV Prevention Research and Global Inequality: Steps Towards Improved Standards of Care. *Journal of Medical Ethics Online* 2005;31:39-47.

"Intensification of poverty and degradation of health infrastructure over recent decades in countries most affected by HIV/AIDS present formidable challenges to clinical research. This paper addresses the overall standard of health care (SOC) that should be provided to research participants in developing countries, rather than the narrow definition of SOC that has characterized the international debate on standards of health care. It argues that contributing to sustainable improvements in health by progressively ratcheting the standard of care upwards for research participants and their communities is an ethical obligation of those in resource-rich countries who sponsor and implement research in poorer ones."

http://jme.bmj.com/cgi/reprint/31/1/39
(accessed 17 April 2008)

Simon C, Mosavel M, van Stade D. Ethical Challenges in the Design and Conduct of Locally Relevant International Health Research. *Social Science and Medicine*, 2007;64(9):1960-1969.

"In this paper, [the authors] consider some of the challenges associated with the ethical need to conduct locally relevant international health research. We examine a cervical cancer research initiative in a resource-poor community in South Africa, and consider the extent to which this research was relevant to the expressed needs and concerns of community members."

http://dx.doi.org/10.1016/j.socscimed.2007.01.009
(accessed 25 August 2008)

Tarantola D, et al. Ethical Considerations Related to the Provision of Care and Treatment in Vaccine Trials. *Vaccine*, 2007, 25:4863-4874.

"Ethical principles of beneficence and justice combined with international human rights norms and standards create certain obligations on researchers, sponsors and public health authorities.[…] However, these obligations are poorly defined in practical terms, inconsistently understood or inadequately applied. The present document addresses specifically the setting of standards applicable to care and treatment in vaccine trials […] and proposes a structured approach to consensual decision making in the context of the clinical trial of vaccines." The paper is based on a series of global consultations initiated by WHO and UNAIDS.

http://dx.doi.org/10.1016/j.vaccine.2007.03.022
(accessed 25 August 2008)

Zong Z. Should Post-trial Provision of Beneficial Experimental Interventions be Mandatory in Developing Countries? *Journal of Medical Ethics*, 2008;34:188-192.

"The need for continuing provision of beneficial experimental interventions after research is concluded remains a controversial topic in bioethics for research….This paper summarises recommendations from international and national guidelines. Ethical principles and practical issues relating to post-trial provision are also discussed. In conclusion, post-trial provision is not necessary in all situations and a set of criteria are proposed to identify the situations that beneficial interventions should be provided beyond the research period. However, mandatory post-trial supply of beneficial experimental interventions should be assured for those who still need and are able to benefit from them but have no alternative access."

http://dx.doi.org/10.1136/jme.2006.018754
(accessed 25 August 2008)

Case 36

Observational study of cervical cancer

> Although this case study is based on research that took place in the 1970s, the questions that it raises remain relevant today.

Cervical cancer causes at least 273 000 deaths globally every year, and about 85% of these deaths occur in developing countries. The incidence of invasive cervical cancer has decreased in countries where women have access to regular Papanicolaou (Pap) smears[1] and subsequent treatment of pre-malignant cervical dysplasias[2] readily available. Most often, women with fatal cases of cervical cancer have never had a Pap smear or have to wait long intervals between Pap screenings.

Cervical dysplasia ranges from low grade squamous intraepithelial lesion (SIL) to high grade SIL.[3] The next stage is carcinoma in situ, indicating that although cancerous cells are present they have not yet spread. In the 1970s, there was lack of consensus in the medical community about which types of dysplasia would progress and become cancerous. Many countries with adequate health facilities took an aggressive position and treated early dysplasia. In many developing countries, however, decisions about when to treat were guided by the belief that not all dysplasias progress to cancer, and this position was supported by previous studies of the natural history of cervical cancer. Thus, in developing countries the most widely accepted stage at which to begin treatment was that of carcinoma in situ, indicating that the cells had become cancerous but remained limited to the cervix.

If doctors could more accurately predict which dysplasias would progress to carcinoma in situ, they could be more specific in deciding which cases to treat early. The development of a more precise diagnostic method that could detect whether a dysplasia was of the type that progresses to cancer would save money and ensure that more women would receive treatment. To design guidelines for a national control programme for cervical cancer, the national medical research council of a South Asian country funded an observational study of cervical cancer to determine which dysplasias were most likely to progress to cancer.

The study, approved by the research ethics committee of the research council, took place over 12 years, beginning in the mid-1970s. Eight government hospitals in one of the country's major cities participated. Most of these hospitals provided both general and specialized gynaecological care but were busy and did not have adequate facilities to manage patients with cancer. Patients with cancer were, therefore, referred to the nearest regional cancer centre for treatment and follow up, with a standard 6-month waiting period to begin treatment.

The researchers elicited the help of community health workers to inform women about the study and encourage them to go to the city hospitals for Pap smears. Women who presented at the eight government hospitals were informed about the study, and were asked to give a Pap smear with informed consent. Since most women in the study were illiterate, the researchers provided information in simple, non-medical language and obtained verbal consent. The researchers did not inform the women that their lesions might progress to cancer. Women were not made aware that treatment was available.

---

[1] A routine screening test used for the detection of early cervical abnormalities, namely precancerous dysplastic changes of the uterine cervix, together with viral, bacterial, and fungal infections of the cervix and vagina. Cervical screening is a relatively simple, low-cost, and non-invasive method. Regular screening for cervical cancer reduces both the mortality from and incidence of cervical carcinoma.

[2] Abnormal development or growth of tissues, organs, or cells. It is the earliest form of precancerous lesion. Dysplasia can be diagnosed as either high or low grade, with high grade dysplasia indicative of a more advanced progression towards malignant transformation.

[3] A general term for the abnormal growth of squamous cells on the surface of the cervix. The changes in the cells are described as low grade (LSIL) or high grade (HSIL), depending on how much of the cervix is affected and how abnormal the cells are. HSIL is regarded as a significant precancerous lesion, whereas low-grade SIL (LSIL) is more benign, since most of these lesions regress.

By the ninth year, researchers had identified more than 1000 women with varying degrees of cervical dysplasia. Women found to have a positive Pap smear at intake were followed up every 3 months, to record the progression of their disorder on the basis of the Pap smear. The end-point for treatment was defined as the development of carcinoma in situ, at which time they were referred to the nearest regional cancer centre, which had a very long waiting list. By the time some of these women were seen by an oncologist, the lesion had progressed to a higher level.

Midway through the study, a leading North American medical journal published the results of a longitudinal study of cervical cancer. The study concluded that cervical dysplasia was a precursor for cervical cancer, and thus that all forms of dysplasia warranted treatment. Despite these new findings, the researchers continued with the study. By the end of the study, 71 women had developed malignancies. In nine of these women, the disease had already spread to other parts of their body. The research team provided no treatment to the women once the study had ended.

Questions

1 Discuss the ethical issues raised by this observational study.

2 Given the shortage of staff, facilities, and equipment in the government-run hospitals, was the medical research council justified in conducting this study? Could national guidelines have been set up without conducting this study?

3 Should continuing services have been offered to participants after completion of the study? If so, what services should have been offered?

4 Does diagnosing a condition or disease during research result in a duty (obligation) to provide care and follow-up for that condition? Is this duty the same whether the condition is diagnosed to include patients in the study or to exclude them?

5 Do the researchers have any responsibility to "take stock" of the situation at least mid-way through such longitudinal studies? Should the sponsors ask for such an evaluation?

6 Should this study have had some stopping rules, or a monitor?

7 Should this study be accepted for publication? If not, how should the results of this study be made generally known to others?

Case 37

Testing a malaria vaccine

A multinational pharmaceutical company has developed a new malaria vaccine that has been successfully tested in Phase I and II trials. The company commissions a team of investigators to conduct a randomized, double-blind, placebo-controlled trial to evaluate the efficacy of the vaccine in combination with the standard immunization scheme. Ultimately, the company's goal is to implement the new vaccine in malaria-prevention programmes. Scientists in an east African country where malaria is endemic express interest in participating in the vaccine research effort. They begin to collaborate with the pharmaceutical company investigators on a study protocol to test the efficacy of the vaccine for reducing malaria-related deaths in the country's children younger than 5 years.

The research team chooses to conduct the study in a southern village where malaria transmission is intense and year-round. In this area, the incidence of clinical malaria rises steeply after the first month of life; the incidence in infants brought to local health facilities with malaria or severe anaemia[1] are 0.7 and 0.6 episodes per child per year, respectively. In this town, a district hospital provides curative health services, while an active maternal and child health (MCH) clinic delivers routine childhood immunizations and offers a monthly weighing clinic. Malaria treatment in the area relies on prompt diagnosis and chloroquine, even though 60% of local parasite strains are resistant to chloroquine.[2]

The researchers plan to recruit participants at the MCH clinic. They will explain the trial to mothers as they bring in their children for first immunization. The clinic nurses agree to assist with translation, but emphasize that they are very busy and might not always be available to aid in this process. To assess each mother's comprehension of the study, the researchers will use a standard set of questions, which are written in the local language. Children of the mothers who provide informed consent will receive a first dose of the vaccine or placebo (aluminium hydroxide) when they present for the first dose of other vaccines provided through the expanded programme on immunization (EPI) at around 1 month of age. Second and third doses will be given at 2 and 7 months of age, respectively.

To monitor the safety of the vaccine, the researchers will examine the children twice in the hour after vaccination, and will document any signs and symptoms of local or systemic reactions. They will further advise parents to return to the clinic if their children experience any health problems such as fever or diarrhoea. Children who develop malaria, as determined by both clinical findings and microscopy, will be treated in the district hospital according to national guidelines (i.e. with chloroquine therapy).

The number of malaria cases will serve as the main study end-point. The researchers will identify cases using a passive case-detection system which has been operating at the district hospital and MCH clinic since 1994 This system will ensure that all participants in the study who attend these health facilities are seen by medical personnel who will provide 24-hour clinical cover.

A few months prior to the proposed start of the trial, the pharmaceutical company's investigators visit the host country to meet with representatives from the department of health to finalize the research protocol. These representatives argue that the informed consent process is inappropriate and does not enable study participants to adequately understand the trial. They note that the female literacy rate is estimated to be below 40%, and that since clinic nurses have a heavy workload, they might not have the time to act as translators. They also request that if the vaccine proves effective, all children in the country should receive free doses of the vaccine for 5 years after completion of the trial.

---

[1] Anemia is a condition in which the haemoglobin concentration in the blood is below a defined level, resulting in a reduced oxygen-carrying capacity of red blood cells. About half of all cases of anaemia can be attributed to iron deficiency; other common causes include infections, such as malaria and schistosomiasis, and genetic factors. The major health consequences include poor pregnancy outcome, impaired physical and cognitive development, increased risk of morbidity in children and reduced work productivity in adults. Pregnant women and children are particularly vulnerable. Anaemia contributes to 20% of all maternal deaths.

[2] Chloroquine has traditionally been used to treat or prevent malaria. Over time, the species of protozoan parasite *Plasmodium falciparum* that causes the worst malaria in humans has developed widespread resistance to chloroquine. *P. falciparum* malaria, which is transmitted by *Anopheles* mosquitoes, is the most dangerous of malaria infections, and causes the highest rates of complications and mortality. It accounts for 80% of all human malarial infections and 90% of deaths. It is more prevalent in sub-Saharan Africa than in other regions of the world. Another species of the protozoan parasite that causes malaria in humans, *P. vivax*, is also transmitted by *Anopheles* mosquitoes. *P. vivax* malaria has fewer complications than *P. falciparum* malaria.

The company's researchers respond that this request is excessive. They explain that the budget for their research cannot cover the cost of vaccinating all 5 million children in the population. They emphasize that they are currently conducting trials for other treatments aimed at the developing country market and it would be unfair to provide free treatment to one country and not to another.

Questions

1. What are the ethical issues raised by this study?

2. Is it appropriate for the researchers to rely on health-centre staff to assist with both translation and assessment of understanding during the informed-consent process?

3. What should be the treatment for those who get malaria?

4. What responsibility, if any, does the company have to the non-study population of the country?

Case 38

Mental health problems of survivors of mass violence

Many developed countries receive a large number of refugees seeking legal asylum. Most of these countries have basic mental health programmes which address the psychological needs of refugees. Most of those programmes, however, are at the local level and in most countries there has been little coherent, nationwide coordination of mental health services with other services for refugees, and virtually no mental health outreach service to refugees and victims of torture. Consequently, the needs of refugees are often misunderstood, and many do not receive the mental health services they need.

A university-based clinic in a European country is pioneering the psychiatric diagnosis and assessment of traumatized populations. Most patients at the clinic are refugees from a South-East Asian country. One dilemma that faces this clinic is that they do not have a well-developed, field-tested method to assess the cultural, political, and social meanings of trauma in the life of civilian populations and the ways in which such experiences alter the everyday lives of the affected individuals. Current diagnostic scales are based on the responses of people from developed countries to trauma, and might not be adequate for measurement of the experiences and reactions of populations that the clinic has to deal with.

The principal researcher at the clinic decides to conduct a study of internally displaced people in the refugees' country of origin. The primary aim is to investigate how social and cultural factors influence the way these internally displaced people react to mass violence and trauma (especially when combined with forced relocation), in order to design a culture-specific diagnostic scale for post-traumatic stress disorder (PTSD).[1] The principal researcher reasons that the knowledge gained from the study on internally displaced people can then be used in the work with the refugees who come to the clinic.

The study will take place in a village that is a 4-hour drive outside the country's capital city. The researchers chose this village as the study site because a large influx of internally displaced people had sought safety there during a violent period of authoritarian rule in the country's history. The local community health centre will serve as the administrative base for the study. A psychiatrist from a large teaching hospital in the capital visits the health centre for one day every month. While at the health centre, he mainly supervises the treatment of chronic psychiatric patients and has no time to engage in long-term psychotherapy or group work with the patients. He has indicated that he does not have the time to be involved with the study.

The European researchers have limited experience in the study country and poor knowledge of the local language. They have therefore decided to recruit community health workers who are well-established in the village to assist them with introductions and translation during the planned home-based interviews. These community health workers, who generally oversee the tuberculosis treatment in the village, will be paid a small honorarium for each house they visit. The researchers will also be accompanied by a group of ethnographers who will collect data on family interactions and social dynamics within the home and village to allow for contextual understanding of the data collected by the researchers. At each house, the researchers will explain the purpose of the study and obtain verbal informed consent for participation.

Each interview will take approximately one hour. The researchers will not record any personal information about the interviewees, who will remain anonymous. The researchers' enquiries will relate to the participants' experiences with violence and trauma, and to the impact of those experiences on their lives.

Based on their professional knowledge and previous experience treating South-East Asian refugees, the researchers will assess each participant's risk for mental illness. Those who are found to be at high risk for mental illness at the time of the interview will be referred to the government health centre for further assessment and treatment. On completion of the study the researchers will provide the study results and their recommendations to the psychiatrist and the ministry of health. No services will be offered as part of the study.

Questions

1. The ethics committee that reviewed this protocol was of the opinion that the survey might cause emotional upset. If you were a member of the ethics committee, would you approve the proposal as submitted? If not, what changes would you ask for and why?

2. What is the risk-benefit analysis of this study? Who will benefit from this study?

3. Guideline 5 of the CIOMS *International Ethical Guidelines for Biomedical Research Involving Human Subjects* http://www.cioms.ch (accessed 9 May 2008) states (in relation to the information that should be provided in an informed consent form) that, after the completion of the study, subjects will be informed of the findings of the research in general, and individual subjects will be informed of any finding that relates to their particular health status. Does this study satisfy the recommendation of this guideline? Why or why not?

4. Should the quality of care at the government clinic to which participants are referred be assessed? Do researchers have a responsibility to upgrade this care? Why or why not?

---

[1] PTSD is an anxiety disorder that can develop after exposure to a terrifying event or ordeal in which grave physical harm occurred or was threatened. Traumatic events that can trigger PTSD include violent personal assaults, natural or human-caused disasters, accidents, or military combat.

Case 39

A longitudinal study of rotavirus incidence among young children

Acute diarrhoeal disease is a leading cause of death in children younger than 5 years in developing countries, and infants younger than 2 years are particularly susceptible. However, few prospective, community-based studies have documented the incidence and cause of diarrhoeal disease among children in Africa. Some hospital-based studies suggest that rotavirus is a major cause of severe diarrhoea in African countries, but the research is not adequate to confirm this belief. The numbers of children affected by and even dying from rotavirus in Africa is, therefore, only an estimate.

A medical university in a West African country has asked a group of epidemiologists from a North American university to work with them to design a longitudinal study of the incidence of rotavirus infection among children younger than 2 years. Since rotavirus is a particular research focus of the North American researchers, they agree to collaborate and offer to fund the study with a grant they have received for rotavirus research.

The study is set in the inner core of a city situated in the tropical zone of sub-Saharan Africa with a population of about 2 million. The inner core comprises the older part of town, which developed without planning and has a high population density. Piped water is unavailable to most residents; therefore, sanitation is poor. The rate of illiteracy and poverty is high, housing is haphazardly constructed, telecommunications are inefficient, and transportation is inadequate.

The study is a prospective, community-based study. A cohort of infants will be selected at birth and followed for 2 years. A sample size of 150 infants has been chosen, based on the reported prevalence of rotavirus and diarrhoea and the workload that the laboratory can conveniently handle.

A general hospital where about 800 babies are delivered every month is chosen as the recruitment centre for the study. The sole inclusion criterion for study participation is residence in the inner core of the city. Pregnant women who are eligible for the study are selected before delivery. Locally recruited research assistants explain the study to mothers in the local language, and informed consent is obtained orally with a witness present. At the time of the birth, cord blood is collected from every infant. Faecal samples are also collected every 3 days until the age of 1 month in order to detect neonatal rotavirus infection. Subsequently, faecal samples are only collected when a child has diarrhoea.

The research assistants do follow-up visits with each child at his or her home on the day of discharge and then every 3 days for the first month of life. Subsequently, the research assistants visit the home of each child every week, and collect data using a standardized questionnaire about illness symptoms. If a child is found to be ill during a home visit, the mother is advised to attend the research clinic the next day, or to attend the local hospital the same day if the illness is considered serious (i.e. fever and vomiting with diarrhoea).

Clinic visits are also required for each child once a month. At each clinic visit the children are treated for any health problems they might have or are referred to specialist clinics at the teaching hospital if necessary. Services provided to the mothers and babies as a means of maintaining participation include:

- Free medical services for the children and members of their family (referral of infants for immunization, referral of mothers to family-planning clinics if they so request, and treatment for older siblings);

- Provision of free anti-malarial prophylaxis to the babies each time they attend the monthly clinic visit; and

- Provision of money to mothers who cannot afford the cost of transport to the clinic (and who might otherwise default).

All of these services will be suspended at the completion of the study. Study results will be presented to the ministry of health – it is hoped that they will influence health-service planning for this disadvantaged part of the city.

Questions

1. How might the provision of free medical services and transport money influence the decision of mothers to enrol their children in this study? How might the provision of free medical services for participants alter the outcomes of the study?

2. Even though this study has a very favourable risk-benefit ratio, it raises an ethical dilemma in relation to the benefits offered. What are the problems with providing extra services during the trial? How can any ill effects be mitigated? Is there any obligation for researchers to continue the extra services after the research is over?

3. Do the investigators have any obligation to follow up with the ministry of health to ensure that the findings have been incorporated into health-service planning?

Case 40

Testing a vaccine for childhood cholera

Cholera is an acute intestinal infection which causes watery diarrhoea. If left untreated, cholera can result very quickly in severe dehydration and even death. The disease is endemic in certain regions of South and South-East Asia, placing young children at high risk of death from a very treatable disease. Oral rehydration therapy (ORT) and intravenous (IV) fluids are very effective for treatment of the fluid losses in cholera, such that mortality from properly treated cases should not exceed 5%. IV fluids cost 50 times more than ORT. Treatment can be carried out in simple treatment centres that are equipped only with cholera cots, buckets, and facilities to provide intravenous fluids if required.

Tetracycline and other appropriate antibiotics reduce the duration of illness by half, but are not essential to treatment. ORT is equally effective for treatment of all dehydrating diarrhoeas. The Cholera and Diarrhoeal Research Institute, a South-East Asian medical research centre, has just received a grant to study the effectiveness of a new vaccine against the cholera strain *Vibrio cholera* 0139, which has recently appeared in two separate regions of the country. The new vaccine was developed at a European university and has been through Phase I and II testing. At the present time the vaccine costs US$ 1.00 per dose; three doses are required. However, this cost is expected to reduce by 75% in the near future. The government's per capita expenditure on health in this region is US$ 5.00 per year.

The field site, a rural rice-growing area with a population of about 75 000, is a 2-hour drive from the medical research centre by mainly country roads. A government clinic services the community, but it is often short on medicines. It has no cholera cots and the physician population changes every 12-18 months. Some traditional practitioners and "unlicenced doctors" work in the area. Few of these providers have modern treatments for cholera or other diarrhoeas.

The vaccine will be given to children who are younger than 5 years in a double-blind fashion: one group will receive the vaccine, and the other a booster dose of tetanus toxoid.[1] As the placebo group is more likely to get cholera, the Institute decides that a treatment facility should be established in the field site to provide state-of-the art care for all patients with cholera and other diarrhoeas. The Institute is prepared to provide the facility, the personnel, the equipment, and medicine free-of-charge to the community. Others suggest that the government clinic ought to be upgraded; but the Institute would have no control over the selection of personnel or quality of care provided at the government clinic. The Institute does not have an endowment and depends on government grants and research awards to finance its activities. Some in the research group are concerned that the Institute risks taking on a long-term commitment to provide treatment that it can not afford.

Questions

1 Who should pay for any long-term health care? What is the Institute's long-term responsibility to provide health care to the community? Should the Institute continue to do so after the study has been completed, or should it provide some support in the future?

2 Should any messages or actions accompany the distribution of vaccines, other than to note all cases of diarrhoea, and to immediately report any that become severe to the treatment facility?

3 If the vaccine is effective, should all participants in the study receive free doses? If so, for how long? Should all other citizens of the country benefit from the results of the study?

---

[1] Tetanus: a disease caused by the bacterium *Clostridium tetani*. It is characterized by muscle spasms, initially in the jaw muscles. As the disease progresses, mild stimuli can trigger generalized tetanic seizure-like activity, which contributes to serious complications and eventually death unless supportive treatment is given. Tetanus can be prevented by the administration of tetanus toxoid, which induces specific antitoxins. To prevent maternal and neonatal tetanus, tetanus toxoid needs to be given to the mother before or during pregnancy, and clean delivery and cord care need to be ensured.

Case 41

Impact of civil war on health systems

Effective control of malaria is heavily dependent on a functioning health care system (i.e. drug distribution, information systems, and preventive, curative, and referral systems). In some of the countries in greatest need of malaria control, however, armed conflict has severely disrupted the structure of their health systems by putting strain on resources and increasing the burden of disease.

A group of researchers from the health ministry of a sub-Saharan African country decide to study the impact of armed conflict on their country's health system, in the hope of identifying interventions that can strengthen health systems in time of war. They decide to collect data from two groups. One group will include those who are most likely to be vulnerable to disease outbreaks during armed conflict, namely, internally displaced people (IDPs) and members of the host communities in which they live. The second group includes key leaders and stakeholders responsible to and for these host communities, such as policymakers, representatives of aid agencies, and officials in charge of health care and of IDP camps. Data from the first group (i.e. vulnerable people) will be collected through focus group discussions while data from the second group (i.e. leaders and stakeholders) will be obtained through semistructured interviews. In order to "purposively select IDP camps and communities that best reflect the reality of the district conflict setting", the IDP camps and communities will be selected by district officials. Focus group participants will be recruited by self-appointed community leaders.

At the end of the study, the researchers plan to hold a 2-day workshop for leaders and officials in charge of health care in each community to present the results. These officials will then be responsible for disseminating the findings to study participants and other members of each community through public meetings. No compensation will be provided to the research participants.

Questions

1. Is it appropriate for community leaders to be responsible for recruitment of participants from a vulnerable population, in this case an internally displaced population?

2. How much is owed to the participants in terms of dissemination of results? If the researchers do not directly convey the findings to participants, is it their responsibility to ensure that health care leaders accurately convey them to participants?

3. Should there be ethical concerns about including both IDPs and members of the host community in the same group? Why or why not?

Case 42

Determining who constitutes the community

An agricultural district in a South Asian country has a population that is 30% tribal. The tribal population of this district comprises 80% of the landless poor in the country, and most live in small hamlets that are 2-3 km from the main village in the district. Only about 10% of the tribal households own land, whereas the non-tribal households have landholdings which provide sustenance but no significant surplus. Recently, because of an irrigation project, even those with small landholdings have been able to substantially raise their incomes by cultivation of fruit and vegetables. Although the daily wages of landless people have increased somewhat, they remain low in proportion to the rise in incomes of the other groups. Over the past decade, tribal people have not been engaged with the local political power structure, and local politics has come to be dominated by farmers with small and medium-sized holdings. These farmers have found willing allies in the large farmers, who belong to the same social class.

Historically, people in this district have used government health services for both primary health care needs and hospital care. The growing private sector has exposed the people to care which is high-tech (although not always appropriate). In the meantime, government services have deteriorated considerably because of lack of investment and the pressure of the growing population. The high cost of private care means that only a small proportion of the population can routinely use private hospital services; the rest still depend on the inadequate and inefficient government system for hospital care.

As part of the health-sector reforms initiated by the state, the health department has been converted into a public-sector company. Its first task is to improve efficiency. To raise funds for improvement of services, it has proposed that hospitals should institute user-charges at a rate which is approximately one third of the fees charged in the private sector for equivalent services. A multilateral agency has been approached for a loan for this project. While the agency agrees in principle with the project's goal, it would like to document people's views about the project through a participatory process. It proposes that in the event of substantial public resistance to the user-fees, some high-tech components of care should be dropped, so that services can continue to be delivered free. Accordingly, the agency directs the health systems corporation to conduct a study to elicit peoples' views about the imposition of user-charges. It provides a standard methodology – the Participatory Rural Appraisal technique – which has been used effectively in Africa.

An external agency is asked to do the study, and decides to conduct focus group discussions with representatives of the community. The protocol guidelines provided suggest that, in each selected village, a committee consisting of one local government body member, the village secretary, the local teacher, and a village elder (or priest) should select participants for the focus group discussions. The protocol stipulates that at least a third of the people in each group should be women. Most of the discussions are held in the community temple in the centre of the main village. Several such focus group discussions are held. The dominant view expressed is that people are willing to pay if the quality of services improves.

During the study, there is an outbreak of gastroenteritis in one of the tribal hamlets in a block where fieldwork is going on. That particular unit of the research team (which consists of young urban professionals) decides to help the staff of the primary health centre, which has sent a mobile unit to the hamlet. When they reach the hamlet, they find that the people are agitated about the unresponsive attitude of the government staff. When the researchers identify themselves, the local leader accuses the research team of conniving with the non-tribal political elite to privatize government services. He shows the team the poverty in which the tribal people live. The team has been unaware of these living conditions because most of their fieldwork has been limited to the main village.

Members of the team review their field notes and notice that fewer than 10% of the participants in their focus group discussions have tribal names; and that most of them are receiving aid from the government (such as loans or development grants for income-generation projects, community schools, or self-help groups). The team reports to their principal investigator, who dismisses their concerns and points out that participants were selected by a very transparent method – with complete community consent, according to an internationally accepted protocol.

Questions

1. Was the method used for selecting participants for the study faulty? If so, what alternative method could have been used? Would that have yielded different results?

2. In a culturally diverse society, with many vulnerable groups who are often minorities, who represents the community? How should representatives be chosen? What obligations does a research team have to ensure that the views of vulnerable groups and minorities are incorporated?

3. In this case, could (and should) the agency include the concerns of the young field workers in its report, and if so, how?

4. What are the obligations of the funders or sponsors with respect to the conduct of the study?

Adapted from a case study contributed by Neha Madhiwalla, Centre for Studies in Ethics and Rights, Mumbai, 2007.

Case 43

Evaluation research on a disability rehabilitation programme

Child-rights groups in a poor democratic country in South Asia have successfully campaigned to make elementary education for all children between the ages of 6 and 14 years a fundamental, justiciable right. The campaign included several groups working in the area of disability, and the resulting law on Right to Education clearly states that it applies equally to all children, including disabled children.

A massive nationwide programme was launched to bring all children aged 6-14 years into the education system. It provides US$ 100 a year for each disabled child. This money is to be disbursed to voluntary organizations to set up appropriate, community-based settings to provide relevant and accessible services for disabled children. Although the programme's primary aim is to improve access to education, organizations can include other service components, such as health (including medical care) and rehabilitation.

Money is allocated between districts based on the recent census, which has, for the first time, covered disabled people. However, since the census data are 5 years old and do not include children whose disability was diagnosed more recently, each organization is also given a one-time grant to survey disability in its area using the same protocol as the census.

The government appoints a well-known public-health expert (who specializes in child health) to evaluate the performance of the programme 3 years after it was launched. A district which is regarded as a model is selected for the study. This evaluation suggests that the programme is efficient and innovative, the commitment of the organizations is evident, and user satisfaction is very high. The district administration is keen to use this study to promote the success of the programme and make it a model for scaling up in the rest of the country.

However, the expert evaluator, who has clinical experience as a paediatrician, is concerned that the evaluation shows that unusually few severely disabled children have been included in the programme. However, repeat surveys using the standard census protocol (including some conducted specifically to check the accuracy of the data collected by the organizations), have yielded similar results.

The expert designs a new protocol, with several probing questions. A pilot survey with this protocol in four poor urban and rural blocks reveals that many severely disabled children (most of whom are bedridden, and unable to care for themselves or communicate verbally), have not been enumerated in any of the surveys or the census. The expert asks some postgraduate medical students to assess these children. They find that the children are being fed and cared for by their parents, but that they do not get medical care or rehabilitation services. Most of them are severely malnourished (e.g. teenagers who weigh less than 15 kg) and several have untreated chronic ailments (including tuberculosis, epilepsy, asthma, and heart defects).

The expert conveys his finding to the programme's district collector, who says that the programme is only obliged to extend services to children identified by the census. Moreover, because the programme already includes more children than the target which is based on the census statistics, their needs exceed the available budget. This administrator appeals to the expert to be more pragmatic, and to refrain from creating a controversy which would not only discredit the programme but also the census, which is the basis on which most government programmes are planned. He points out that inclusion of disabled children would divert resources away from children with better chances of leading productive lives. However, he expert argues that he has a responsibility to reveal that the research data are systematically biased.

Questions

1. The researcher feels a responsibility to reveal the truth, which is a key ethical concern for research as an enterprise of knowledge creation. Would he be justified in insisting that the information should be made public, even though no action (in terms of services or care for the severely disabled children) might result from it?

2. Should the design of this evaluation study have been reviewed by an ethics committee? Why or why not?

3. Who is most at "risk" during the conduct of health systems evaluation studies? How can the "risk" to health care professionals be decreased during the conduct of these evaluations?

Contributed by Neha Madhiwalla, Centre for Studies in Ethics and Rights, Mumbai, India, 2007.

Case 44

Clinical benefits of an immune-modifying supplement in HIV therapy

In 1995, two professors from prominent North American universities organized the largest randomized drug trial of the past decade in HIV-infected people. With a nationwide team of investigators, they evaluated the clinical benefits of an immune-modifying drug that was intended to supplement standard treatments for HIV. Their working hypothesis was that the drug could boost the immune system's response to HIV. The trial was funded by a pharmaceutical company that entered into a pre-study agreement with the researchers. The agreement stated that the company had complete ownership of the data, but that ownership would not restrict the researchers' ability to publish their study results.

For the clinical trial, the researchers enrolled more than 2500 HIV-infected patients at 77 medical centres in the United States of America. Most of these patients were already receiving antiretroviral therapies, and none had ever developed the major clinical characteristics associated with the progression of HIV infection to clinical AIDS. Half of the patients received the experimental drug plus standard treatment, and the other half received standard treatment only. The primary measures of the drug's efficacy were the quantity of the virus in the blood, T-cell counts, and bodyweight. The secondary measure was progression to AIDS or death.

The study was terminated 5 months early, in May 1999, after an analysis by an independent data monitoring board showed that the compound had no clinical benefit and that it would be unlikely that the study, if continued, would conclude otherwise. The principal researchers agreed with this decision and the study was stopped.

The researchers presented the results of the study to the pharmaceutical company. After conducting their own analyses, the company announced that they had found a sign that the compound was active. The company then issued a statement, with which the researchers did not agree, about the positive effect of the drug on viral load.

Contrary to the provisions of the pre-study agreement and the research contract, the company refused to provide the final data unless the researchers agreed to include additional analyses specified by the company in any publications. The company also insisted upon being allowed to review and approve (or disapprove) all publications. The researchers believed these terms to be unacceptable and decided to write a paper based on the data then available to them, which they estimated to be 95% of the total cases. The paper was published in a prestigious, peer-reviewed medical journal.

The researchers believed that the results of this trial were important not only to the doctors and patients enrolled in the trial, but also to the investigators of other trials of the same drug. At the time, one other study of this drug had been completed and two others were being planned. A clinical trial funded by a national research institute using this experimental drug to treat AIDS was stopped soon after this publication.

The pharmaceutical company filed a lawsuit against the university that employed the principal researcher on the study. The university filed a counter-claim, arguing that its researcher had the right to publish industry-sponsored research findings that might be unfavourable or neutral.

Questions

1 Who owns the data from a study? Do sponsors of research have the right to prevent dissemination and publication of research results for any reason? Under what circumstances would sponsors have this right?

2 Was the decision of the researchers to publish the results of their study correct, in your view?

3 Assume that an investigator has agreed not to publish unless the sponsor first gives approval. The findings from the study indicate that the drug is harmful for treatment of a certain condition. The sponsor does not give approval for publication. What can or should the investigator do?

Case 45

Genetic research on an island population

An island nation has a population of about 90 000, all of whom are of a single ethnic background. There is little or no immigration to the island and hence the genetic make-up of the population is quite homogenous. This presumed genetic homogeneity along with the high incidence of certain diseases in the population are seen as an advantage by some researchers who are looking for specific alleles associated with polygenic diseases.

The island's government is a monarchy, although it also includes a prime minister and a cabinet, a third of which is chosen by popular vote. A popular movement has been pressing for more democratic representation and a free press in the country. Most of the islanders belong to one of the several denominations of Christianity that spread during the active missionary movements led by European colonizers during their 100-year presence on the island, which ended 30 years ago.

The island's economy is supported by a narrow base of agricultural exports and some tourism. The GDP is approximately US$ 1500 per person. Most food is imported and unemployment is about 15%. Literacy is almost universal, and health services are reasonably good and free. A growing concern, however, is the rising rate of diabetes and obesity; 18% of the population is estimated to have diabetes, which is twice the prevalence reported 25 years ago. Changes in diet and physical activity, including increased consumption of imported fatty foods overlaid on a possible genetic predisposition for the disease, are believed to account for the rising prevalence of diabetes.

In 2001, after negotiations with the government, a European biotechnology firm announced an agreement to conduct genetic research designed to identify disease-related genes in the relatively isolated and homogeneous island population. The company planned to target families with members who had already been diagnosed with diabetes for sampling and genetic analysis. A newspaper account in Europe described the arrangement as allowing the company "exclusive rights" to collect blood samples from the islanders, provided that islanders gave individual informed consent for genetic analysis. In fact, the word "exclusive" does not appear in the agreement.

The company has made a commitment to donate a certain amount of money to the country's ministry of health, including plans to construct a new research centre on the island, and to share some portion of any royalties generated by commercial products either developed for the project or as a result of it.

The agreement, first announced in the European press, was immediately criticized by the island's community groups. The head of the popular democracy movement stated several objections, including a lack of public discussion of the project; inadequate transparency on the part of the government about its actions; a failure to consider the privacy of those whose family members might participate in the project on the basis of individual consent; opposition to the notion of patenting DNA and other life forms; and the lack of guarantees of any benefits either for those who participate in the study or for the island population more generally. In addition, he contended that the benefits would be minimal compared with the material gain that might be realized by the company in attracting new capital and producing successful products. At the time, the country had no existing intellectual-property law or regulation of biological research, and thus had a limited ability to protect its own interests.

The island's organization of Christian churches published a statement in a journal of medical ethics that opposed the project on the basis of religious beliefs, namely that patenting of "life forms" was a violation of respect for the sanctity of life and fundamental religious principles. Shortly after the protests, the company withdrew its plans for the project and pursued agreements to gather samples elsewhere.

Questions

1. Does a group of people have collective ownership of their genetic heritage? If so, how could this ownership be defined?

2. What ethical concerns arise about the ability of national governments to negotiate and decide agreements for genetic research in their populations?

3. How can benefit-sharing arrangements be evaluated in terms of fairness, transparency, and responsiveness to national needs?

4. How can it be determined that benefits that might accrue to a body or governmental organization in the country best serve the interests of the population?

5. Would it have made any difference to the ethical implications if the genetic research project was carried out by a non-profit entity, as opposed to a for-profit commercial entity?

Chapter VII

Privacy and Confidentiality

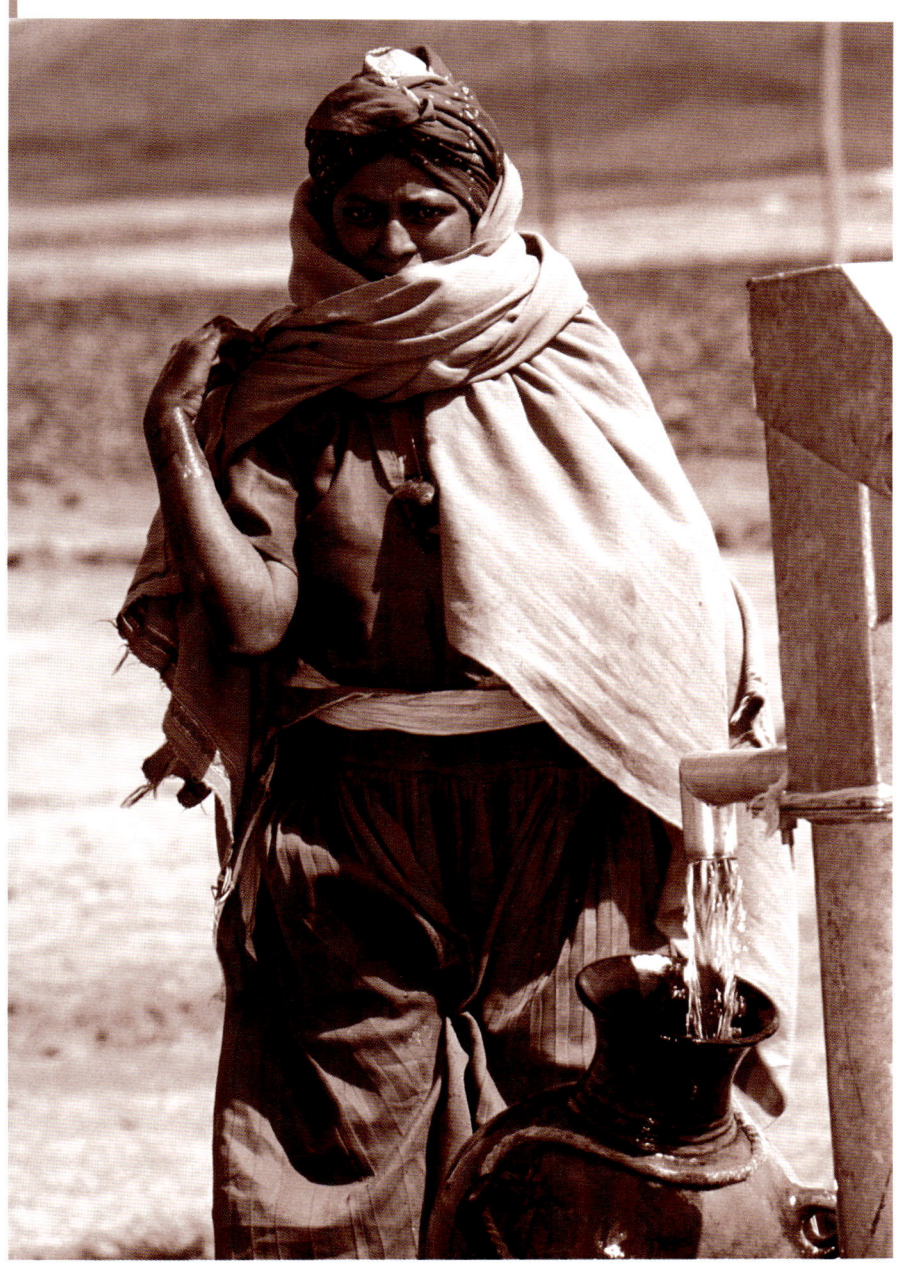

© WHO

Introduction: Chapter VII

Who controls access to information?

Privacy and confidentiality – the first an interest or right of either individuals or small groups of people, and the second a duty of professionals – might be jeopardized by health research. When privacy and confidentiality can be fully protected without the scientific value of the research being compromised, scientists clearly have a duty to do so, barring specific obstacles. In some cases, conflicts between the interests of science and participants' interests in privacy and confidentiality cannot be fully resolved. Although the default position favours protection of participants in these instances, a REC may need to establish how seriously participants' interests would be compromised by a research project, and to weigh these potential risks against the value of the knowledge to be gained. To identify the interests at stake and to estimate the likelihood and extent of any potential harm, the REC needs to consider what privacy and confidentiality consist of and why they are valuable.

Defining the interests at stake in a research project

Privacy is difficult to define in a non-circular way. What is private *is* personal or sensitive, but these terms are really synonyms for private. Privacy interests are often grouped into three categories:

1. Control over who has access to information about someone (e.g. whether they have the gene for a serious, adult-onset disease). This control extends not only to which people have access to the information, but also how much access individuals are willing to provide to others, and when and under what circumstances they are willing to do so;

2. Control over who has the right to observe someone when they are not in a public space (e.g. a doctor might be allowed to examine someone medically, but others who might have a legitimate interest in observing that examination, such as medical trainees or researchers might not);

3. Control over specific decisions concerning oneself (e.g. women's decisions about whether to have children).

Privacy issues in research that are associated with human patients usually involve the first category and, in the context of observational studies, occasionally the second. The third category mainly involves the extent to which the state can restrict individual choices about matters that are especially important to people's control over their lives. The word privacy is sometimes used to refer to what an individual would like to keep from others and, in other instances, to what the individual has a right to keep from others. For example, people who have been convicted of crimes might hope that none of their associates learn about previous legal problems, but these facts are typically a matter of public record.

The definition of what is perceived as an infringement of privacy varies from culture to culture and should be taken into consideration. For people living in developed countries, the premium placed on the individual and the boundaries of the individual is very high. However, in some cultures, people would be concerned or even alarmed if told that routine information related to health care was confidential and would not be shared with their family members. They might also start to wonder why the researchers were being so secretive and might become wary of the research process. RECs should be cognizant of these differences and judiciously apply the requirements of privacy and confidentiality in research, especially when no tangible harms from research can accrue.

Confidentiality involves fulfilment of an obligation not to disclose private information. The obligation usually arises within a relationship in which it is necessary to share information with someone who would not otherwise be privy to it (e.g. when a patient tells her doctor that she has had a previous abortion). In most countries, doctors have pledged not to repeat information that they have learned from patients because the profession sees confidentiality as essential, not only for successful health care, but more importantly to protect the trust that is placed in doctors by their patients.

Tangible and intangible interests

Privacy and confidentiality protect information of tangible value to individuals. A mother might dread a forthcoming counseling session with her child's geneticist, fearing that her husband will learn for the first time that he is not the child's father, and that this knowledge will adversely affect her life and that of her child. To provide a second example, if it were known that a man has inherited the gene for Huntington's disease (a progressively disabling and lethal neurological disorder), he might be refused a position for which the employer would need to invest in substantial training, and he would also probably be unable to obtain life insurance because of the likelihood that he would become disabled in mid-life and die prematurely.

Privacy and confidentiality also apply when an individual has no such tangible interests at stake. People might tell a physician specific intimate details about themselves but would feel shame if strangers overheard the conversation. Even if people's opinions about sensitive moral or political issues, or details about the manner in which they live, are conventional, they ordinarily disclose these opinions only to intimates or to others with whom they are in relationships of trust.

Control over who might know intimate facts about people and who might view people in private protects individuality. Nearly all societies enforce conventions about how people act, talk, and appear. At home, away from the public's gaze, people can be themselves – that is, act as they choose without regard to social conventions. Protection of privacy helps to provide an opportunity for personal development by allowing people to behave in different ways when they need not be concerned with keeping up appearances or meeting the expectations of others.

Control over who might perceive people in different contexts, and who might know about their personal lives, allows distinctions between the types of relationships that people have. Individuals might confide in their spouses and other intimates what they keep from good friends; mere acquaintances might be told less. Enforcing obligations of confidentiality on doctors (and other professionals) aims to create relationships in which people can share very personal information with someone with whom they do not otherwise have a close connection. An obligation of confidentiality is not obviously inherent in the relationship between a researcher and a research participant, rather, the obligation is created because it is essential for participants to feel confidence that the data they provide to a researcher will remain private if researchers are going to be able to collect not only information that is usually private but that also includes details about intimate areas of life – e.g. studies on sexual risk behaviours, drug dependence, or socioeconomic status. Hence, research participants need to be aware not only of this obligation, but also of the extent to which this confidentiality will (or will not) be maintained.

Identifying the intangible interests protected by duties of privacy and confidentiality is a difficult task. Without considering these interests, accounting for the value of privacy is difficult, especially when no tangible injury is risked. However, although no tangible harms might exist, invasion of privacy or breaches of confidentiality nevertheless constitute wrongs. These wrongs should be avoided in research even when no harms can be shown and RECs should bear this notion in mind. At the same time, the significance of privacy should not be exaggerated. A researcher can learn a great deal about participants, including perhaps some information that they would prefer no one to know, without actually causing them harm.

Challenges in balancing personal and societal interests

Many societies restrict personal control over specific information and over the ability to control perceptions, even when people might strongly wish to retain power over such information. Perceptive individuals can learn a lot about others by watching how they dress and talk in public; for example, a shopkeeper or a detective might be able to judge whether someone is lying. Public records can provide personal information about people from automobile registration information to business or professional licenses. For that reason, research that involves private information obtained through public sources presents a particular challenge to RECs.

Debates about privacy and confidentiality in health research are bound to become more contentious in the future. The advent of the electronic medical record, the growth of genetic databanks and other large repositories of medical information for research and administration of health care, and the ease of linking databases suggest the start of a regime in which individuals lose the ability to control what others might know about their health and their lives generally. When personal genome maps become inexpensive, a development that is only a few years away, a wealth of information about individuals will become available and can be linked to other data. The genome identifies the individual permanently (and largely unchangeably), and furthermore provides strong identifiers for relatives and descendants.

Some of these same developments offer potential benefits of great value to individuals and societies. For example, genetic databanks are already allowing researchers to uncover genetic predispositions to serious diseases. An improved understanding of the social determinants of health can be derived through the analysis of great quantities of survey data. Adverse events can be linked to new pharmaceutical drugs long after initial approval. All these advances might be slowed or blocked if controls on access or use of identifying information, which are put in place to protect privacy and confidentiality, are too strong. This is a particular concern if the threat to a privacy interest is slight or merely theoretical, and the potential value of the research is great. Absolute priority for privacy and confidentiality can be as much an error as insufficient regard for these interests.

Role of RECs in assessment of privacy and confidentiality

Given the importance of privacy and confidentiality, RECs must assess that privacy concerns have been adequately dealt with and that the information obtained from research participants is dealt with confidentially. To achieve this aim, RECs should focus on: how and where the contact with potential participants will be made and information gathered; whether others will be present; how identifiable information will be gathered; whether participants will be comfortable in the setting in which information is obtained; whether the procedures for identification of individuals minimize the invasion of privacy; and how information will be stored, for how long, in what form, and with whom it will be shared. For example, participants might not wish to be seen entering a counselor's office if the counselor is known to provide counseling on sexually transmitted infections, and investigators need to consider ways of protecting the privacy of research participants in such a situation.

However, research investigators may be legally bound to disclose some information (even if it is obtained on the premise of confidentiality) to relevant authorities or organizations, for example if investigators identify cases of child abuse or violence against women, they might be statutorily required to report these to the police; if prospective criminal activities are disclosed to a researcher, he or she could have legal (and moral) duties to warn or protect third parties; or a court might subpoena a researcher to hand over records in research on illegal activities, sex work, or drug use. Researchers in most countries do not enjoy legal privileges or protection from subpoenas or disclosure that is ordered by the courts. Therefore when designing studies in which there is a a risk that disclosure will be required, the investigator needs to consider these issues very carefully and warn research participants of such possibilities when appropriate.

Privacy is not a concern of an individual alone – communities might sometimes need to keep some information about the group as a whole from becoming public; and in certain circumstances some could be stigmatized just because they agreed to take part in research. In some contexts, publication of the exact site of a study could be harmful, even though individuals are not named (e.g. individuals from a community in which HIV seroprevalence was studied might be discriminated against by employers or by prospective marriage partners because the district came to be incorrectly assumed to be a high prevalence area for HIV). Such social stigmatization can often be long term, with long lasting harmful effects, and both investigators and RECs should be especially aware of this possibility and take all precautions to avoid it.

Suggested readings

Shalowitz DI, Miller FG. Disclosing Individual Results of Clinical Research. *Journal of the American Medical Association*, 2005; 294(6):737-740.

This paper discusses the responsibility of investigators to communicate the results of research to study participants. The author argues that "disclosure of individual results should be addressed in all research involving human participants."

http://jama.ama-assn.org/cgi/content/full/294/6/737
(accessed 9 May 2008)

Lawlor DA, Stone T. Public Health and Data Protection: An Inevitable Collision or Potential for a Meeting of Minds? *International Journal of Epidemiology*, 2001; 30:1221-1225.

This paper reviews current data protection legislation and guidance, looking at its consequences on public health practices. In addition, it discusses recent changes to legislation and guidance in relation to established medical principles.

http://ije.oxfordjournals.org/cgi/content/full/30/6/1221
(accessed 9 May 2008)

Case 46

Studying Nevirapine in West Africa

A study in a West African country is designed to examine the effectiveness of the antiretroviral drug, Nevirapine, when administered to HIV-positive women during labour and then to their newborns for the first three months after birth. The aim of the study is to assess whether Nevirapine can reduce the perinatal transmission of HIV infection in infants aged younger than one year.

Pregnant women have their blood drawn and tested for HIV in the latter stages of pregnancy. They are assured that their test results will be kept confidential, as will any other treatment they receive. If they are HIV-positive, they are offered Nevirapine, which will be administered just before birth and for three days afterwards.

One of the women who tests positive is the fourth wife of an older man. She discloses to the physician that she has had sexual relations with two men from the community during the past year. The doctor who has taken the history is concerned that the husband could contract HIV from his wife and pass it to his other wives. The doctor tells the woman that she should inform her husband, but she insists that nothing be said since he would certainly throw her out of the house and might even physically harm her. The doctor tells his colleagues that he feels compelled to tell the husband. Some agree and others feel that the confidentiality promised at the beginning of the study must be honoured.

Questions

1. Should the husband and/or the two other men be told? What reasoning leads you to your conclusion?

2. Are there any situations where the promise of confidentiality should not be honoured?

3. Does the researcher or physician have an obligation to develop or discuss a safety plan with the woman about whether or not the information on HIV status should be shared?

Case 47

The quality of care in a family welfare programme[1]

A group of university-based investigators undertake an evaluation of the quality of care in a family welfare programme in one of the states of a South Asian country. The project is funded by a grant from a European university to the South Asian university which employs the researchers. As part of the evaluation process, the investigators plan to interview the doctors, supervisors, and multipurpose health workers employed at selected primary health centres (PHCs) in the state, and the family-planning clients who visit those PHCs. Client-provider interactions at the centres, and at a sterilization camp organized by one of the selected PHCs, will be observed for one week.

An ethical review board, convened to advise the project, and consisting of leading researchers in the country, recommended that all information that could lead to the identification of specific PHCs by those in authority should be specifically avoided. Even mentioning a political division (population 20 000) in which the study was undertaken could result in repercussions to the PHC or its employees, all of whom are employees of the state, by the national or state government health programmes. Therefore, the board has recommended that investigators should not collect any information which could later be used by authorities to identify specific PHCs or employees. If the information was absolutely necessary to the study, it should be carefully disguised to preserve anonymity.

The investigators requested permission for the study from the state government, as the operator of the PHCs and the employer of the staff. Health officials from the national and state governments reviewed the proposal and approved the project, including its consent documentation and other necessary steps designed to protect the confidentiality of the PHCs and health workers.

The study began on time and without incident. During week four of the study, however, a field researcher who was observing procedures at a local PHC noticed a health worker reusing syringes. This practice creates the risk of spreading infection between clients. Without mentioning names, the researcher reported the incident to the health worker's supervisor, who thanked her and assured her that the situation would be rectified.

A week later, the field researcher returned to the clinic to deliver some papers. Out of curiosity, she stopped at the outpatient area of the clinic, where she once again observed health workers reusing syringes. Although the field researcher knew that the project had guaranteed confidentiality to the clinic and its workers, she was concerned that the clinic had apparently done nothing to correct this problem. Unsure what to do, she asked the principal investigator for guidance.

Questions

1 Should the principle of confidentiality be strictly upheld?

2 Should the principal investigator undertake any action? If so, what should it be?

3 What advice should the principal investigator give to the field researcher?

---

[1] This case study is very similar to Case Study 48 and raises similar, but slightly different issues.

Case 48

Responding when study findings are challenged[1]

A team of university researchers have completed an evaluation of the quality of care in a family welfare programme of a state in a South Asian country. The researchers complied with the recommendations of a research ethics committee that they should ensure the confidentiality of all identifying data about the primary health centres (PHCs) – which deliver the programme – and their employees: all information which could later be used by authorities to identify specific PHCs or employees has been made anonymous or disguised. The state and national governments had also reviewed the proposal and approved the project, including the provisions for the confidentiality of the PHCs and health workers. Upon completion of the study, the researchers presented their results at a dissemination workshop in the state capital which was attended by health activists, bureaucrats from the health ministry at the national and state levels, and health officials.

The investigators reported their findings that the quality of services provided by the PHCs was widely distributed along a bell-curve: some PHCs were doing an excellent job but others were not. They reported that no special efforts had been made to maintain a consistent, high standard of care, and that national-level protocols for service delivery were absent. In particular, when some of the PHCs organized sterilization camps, accommodation for clients had been given minimal consideration, and water and sanitation facilities were insufficient to meet clients' needs. The large number of clients sterilized in a short period of time at some camps also violated accepted medical protocols.

After the study's conclusions were reported, the officials and government representatives asked the investigators to identify the PHCs. The researchers refused to do so, pointing out that the government had agreed that the results should be anonymized when it approved the study.

The government officials then argued that the investigators had fabricated their evidence, and denied that such adverse conditions could exist. The officials said that the confidentiality agreement did not apply, since it was designed to protect PHCs and workers against discipline or retribution, whereas they only wanted to have the identity of the PHCs and staff revealed so they could verify the study findings and, if necessary, institute appropriate policies and practices.

Questions

1 Should the names of the PHCs be given to the state (or national) government and/or the health officials, in order to allow them to verify the accuracy of the findings, or for any other reasons?

2 How valid is the argument that if something is to be done to improve conditions in the PHCs and the health camps run by them, then the PHCs that are performing poorly must be identified?

3 Under what circumstances (if any) should promises of confidentiality be ignored?

---

[1] This case study is very similar to Case Study 47 and raises similar, but slightly different issues.

Case 49

Determining post-abortion complication levels

An eastern European country has passed a law to make abortion legal for a range of social and medical indications. Nevertheless, legal abortion centres are neither geographically accessible, nor always functioning effectively. Indeed, abortions outside of the legally recognized sector are still estimated to occur between two and five times more frequently than do those in legally recognized centres.

Although the demographic profile of abortion-seekers, the dangers associated with illegal abortions, and the links between abortion and fertility control have been well documented, much of the evidence has come from studies in urban hospitals and clinics, many of which relied on reviews of hospital records rather than primary sources. Because of their self-selective nature, even well-designed hospital studies cannot adequately address issues such as why women would choose a legally recognized centre or not, and the consequences of those choices for their experiences of abortion, including post-abortion complications. The few community-based studies mostly take the form of knowledge, attitude, and practice surveys, which have problems of deliberate under-reporting and inadvertent classification of induced abortions as spontaneous events.

To determine the rate of complications after abortions and determine their correlation to the provider-type, a local non-governmental research group have designed a study with both qualitative and quantitative approaches. The group aims to examine women's choice of provider, their abortion experiences, and consequences. The study covers 140 villages (population 320 000) in an area where government abortion services are provided through the district hospital, some rural hospitals, and a few primary health care centres. In addition to these facilities in the public sector, several small private hospitals and some non-governmental organizations (NGOs) offer various legally recognized abortion services.

During a three-month preparatory phase, key informants in the community and at abortion centres were interviewed about the range of providers and areas of concern to the community and providers. The study team proposed to find cases of abortion in the study area both from community-based health workers and women's groups and from health care providers in the formal and informal sectors who provide abortion services.

All health care providers who perform abortions and who agree to be part of the case-finding process are given an instruction sheet about the purpose and methods of the project. They discuss the project with abortion-seekers and obtain consent from those who are willing to be interviewed at home by the research team. Oral consent is obtained since some participants are illiterate. Health care providers are not offered incentives for recruiting participants, and they are not required to inform researchers about the people who refuse to be interviewed. Community-based health workers and women's groups within the community are asked to schedule interviews between the researchers and consenting abortion-seekers who have not been identified by the facility-based system. Interviewers go to the villages of those who have had an abortion no more than 3 months after the procedure.

Study participants are to be enrolled prospectively over an 18-month study period. To protect women from possible stigma associated with abortion, participation in the study will be disguised as follows:

- Interviews with women who are known to have had an abortion will only be conducted if several of these women live in a community, and dummy interviews using the same questionnaire will be conducted with other women in the village who are not known to have had an abortion.

- The interview will focus on gynaecological problems, past pregnancy outcomes, and health complications, rather than on the abortion episode.

- A team of interviewers will created artificial privacy during the interview; one person will conduct the interview while the others engage family members in dummy interviews.

- Women will be free to discontinue their interviews at any time without prejudice.

The study is submitted to an international foundation, which agrees to fund it. After its approval by the state review committee, the study is presented to the funder's research ethics committee. All but one member of the committee, who is an anthropologist who has worked extensively in the rural parts of that country, approve the study. The anthropologist is concerned that the confidentiality of abortion-seekers could be compromised, and wants assurances that the records that identify each research participant will be kept confidential. The leader of the research group responds that all records will be kept under lock and key in the main offices of the NGO, which is nowhere near the study site.

Questions

1. Does the process for identification of women who have had an abortion by using community and women's groups and formal and informal health workers as information sources properly ensure confidentiality?

2. Should oral consent substitute for written consent in a population in which illiteracy is common and people are reluctant to put any signature or identifying mark on a written document that they might not understand?

3. Will the interview process adequately protect privacy? Comment on the procedures that are designed to protect the women who had consented to be interviewed at the time they underwent an abortion (dummy interviews in the community, clustering of interviews, and dummy interviews with other family members during the interview with the woman).

4. What additional measures might be used to protect interviewees from the possibility of unwanted attention?

5. Is this method of recruitment of "abortion seekers" appropriate and free of coercion?

Case 50

Evaluating the cost-benefit ratio of long-term care services

The mental health institute of a Central American country has historically offered financial support to community mental health centres (CMHCs) that provide care for people who have severe, chronic mental illness (including most individuals with schizophrenia, and many who suffer from manic-depressive illness and chronic major depression). The institute has given this support in the form of reimbursements to CMHCs for long-term care services, which typically include supervision of medications and, in some cases, transportation to doctors' appointments.

The institute has recently implemented a research programme aimed at ensuring that the CMHCs offer high-quality, cost-effective care. A study is designed that will use outcome measures (for example, number of admissions to hospitals per year) to compare the cost and benefit of long-term care services with the provision of medications without these supportive services (i.e. without supervison, transportation to appointments). To this end, the institute will gather demographic and clinical information from the confidential psychiatric records of individuals who receive long-term care services.

Recognizing that individual consent is required for release of this sensitive information, the institute has contacted the CMHCs and instructed clinicians to obtain such consent from patients who currently receive long-term care services. The institute has also informed the CMHCs that reimbursement for such services will henceforth only be provided for patients who have signed consent forms agreeing to this release of information.

Some CMHC clinicians object to the institute's actions, arguing that a government agency should not have direct access to people's confidential mental health records, and that the government's plan to withhold reimbursement for individuals who do not provide consent amounts to coercion.

Representatives of the institute have responded that the state needs access to this information in order to perform outcomes research. In fact, the institute for mental health argues, the net result of such data gathering will be an improvement in services to the chronically ill. These benefits, they say, will outweigh any theoretical disadvantage such individuals might experience as a result of sharing their confidential records.

Questions

1 Under what circumstances is it ethically acceptable for a state agency to have access to individual medical records? Are those circumstances satisfied in this study?

2 Even if signature on consent forms from the recipients of long-term care services had been obtained, what other conditions would need to be satisfied for it to be a valid consent?

3 If you were a member of a research ethics committee evaluating this project, what advice would you give to ensure that the project was conducted ethically?

Case 51

Research on an identifiable population

A team of molecular biology researchers wishes to study the basis of alcoholism in selected native peoples of North America. This research is based on reports of a significant correlation between alcoholism and several forms of brainwave activity that are measurable by electroencephalography: Caucasian and African Americans with these brainwave patterns have a higher risk of alcoholism. There is also some evidence of a genetic linkage between the brainwaves and traits of alcoholism.

Since the prevalence of alcoholism is high in many North American indigenous tribes, this research team believes it is important to ascertain whether there is a genetic linkage between brainwave patterns and alcoholism in this population. The researchers propose to select 300 families which have high incidences of alcoholism. Compensation to research participants will average US$ 300 for two days of participation. A preliminary survey in the tribal communities indicates that many hundreds of individuals are interested in participating.

A week before the research ethics committee was to meet to review the protocol, the committee's chair received the following memorandum from a representative body for the selected community:

"The [XXX] tribal community urges the Research Ethics Committee to reject this study. No tribal community or representative body has been contacted to discuss the concerns that our members might have with the study. This oversight fails to recognize our community's legitimate concerns about how the information this may produce will be used scientifically and whether the methods used are in keeping with our religious and cultural values. For example, the research plan does not describe how blood samples will be treated. Like most indigenous communities, the [XXX] Tribe traditionally considers all parts of the body sacred, including materials derived from the body (such as blood products or organs). Of equal concern, we believe that both our community as a whole and individuals within the community may be stigmatized by the proposed research. We point to the history of discrimination and stigmatization that has burdened our people, particularly in relation to alcoholism, as proof of this concern. Since this study offers no immediate benefits and poses significant risk, it should not be approved."

Questions

1 In view of the memo from the representative body should the research ethics committee ignore the results of the preliminary survey that indicates that many individuals are interested in participating in the survey? How can such committees evaluate whether representative bodies truly represent the community? Should the representative body speak for individuals?

2 How should the research ethics committee respond? Should it approve the protocol, and if so, under what conditions?

3 What modifications could be made to the protocol that might address the concerns raised?

Based on a case of the same title provided by the National Institute for Human Genome Research.

Case 52

Case-control study of vasectomy and prostate cancer

Epidemiologists in an industrialized country propose to investigate the association between vasectomy and adenocarcinoma[1] of the prostate gland, using a case-control study design. Men with prostate cancer, confirmed by histological examination, will be identified through their clinicians' records. The control group, consisting of men of similar ages who do not have prostate cancer, will be chosen at random from the national election registry. Since the country in question has good telephone services, the investigators propose to conduct the study by telephone interviews and to complete the data-collection questionnaires using the information provided in these telephone interviews.

Interviewers will contact all eligible participants by telephone to seek their consent to take part in the study. However, because the researchers believe that participants' responses could be biased if they knew the objective of the study – namely to investigate the possible association between vasectomy and prostate cancer – participants will not be told the precise nature of the study but only that they are being invited to take part in a study of risk factors for prostate disease.

The questions to be asked of both the men with prostate cancer and the control group will cover variables believed to be associated with this type of prostate cancer (e.g. age, marital status, number of children, history and time since vasectomy, previous and concurrent illnesses, use of medical services, personal history of smoking and alcohol consumption, use of other fertility regulation methods, and family history of prostate cancer).

Questions

1 Is it ethically acceptable to gain access to the medical records of these patients without first asking their permission? Why or why not?

2 Is it acceptable to do this type of study by telephone interview? Why or why not?

3 Since the study will be conducted by telephone questionnaire, written informed consent will not be possible. Is this acceptable?

4 The premise (and purpose) of the study will not be revealed to the subjects. If you think that this is not acceptable, how would you answer the participants' argument that revealing the premise would result in invalid results because the responses would be biased?

---

[1] An adenocarcinoma is a malignant tumour that originates in glandular (secretory) tissue.

Case 53

Studying health-seeking behaviour

A team of social scientists concerned with improvement of women's health wants to learn why women do not return to the hospital for the results of Papanicolaou (Pap) tests.[1] They have a research project to follow up with women who have a presumptive diagnosis of cervical cancer (a positive Pap test) but who do not return to the hospital, as advised, to receive their test results. The aim of the research is to find out how to improve services to these women.

The chiefs of service in the hospital grant permission to the social scientists to conduct their investigations. Physicians provide the researchers with access to hospital records from which the researchers obtain the names and addresses of the patients. They then visit the patients in their homes. The social scientists identify themselves as researchers and ask permission to interview the patients in their homes. They then interview those patients who consent and give them information about the results of their Pap test.

The researchers inform the women that they should return to the hospital for follow-up care. They facilitate this process by giving the women the names of physicians that they can go to directly, thereby enabling them to avoid the usual bureaucratic obstacles. They defend their methodology by stating (1) that the study offers women health benefits; (2) that the study facilitates more rapid and easy access for women to the appropriate health services; and (3) that patients' records in public hospitals belong to the hospital and not to patients. Furthermore, the study is likely to reveal information that will enable the hospital to improve its services to women by effecting better follow-up, thereby reducing the rate of cervical cancer.

Questions

1. Is it justified for the chiefs of service to grant permission to the social scientists to use the records without the consent of the patients? Is confidentiality breached?

2. Is it appropriate that the investigators visit the patients at their residence without permission?

3. Should social scientists provide the results of the Pap test to the patients?

4. In what other way could the investigators have approached the problem?

Adapted from material developed by the UNDP/UNFPA/WHO/World Bank Special Programme of Research, Development and Research Training in Human Reproduction, Bangkok Thailand, 2004.

---

[1] A routine screening test used for the detection of early cervical abnormalities, namely precancerous dysplastic changes of the uterine cervix, together with viral, bacterial, and fungal infections of the cervix and vagina. Cervical screening is a relatively simple, low cost and non-invasive method. Regular screening for cervical cancer reduces both the mortality and incidence of cervical carcinoma.

Case 54

Health promotion survey research on a commercial farm

A large farm in southern Africa recruits both men and women as seasonal labourers from the nearby town, local villages and other rural areas. The male-female ratio among the seasonal labourers is approximately four to one, although other women are involved informally in the economy of the farm selling vegetables, game meat, tea, wine, and beer to farm workers in and around the farm. Most of the women employed as seasonal workers are younger than 25 years, and 70% are single.

Only some of the seasonal workers actually live in the farm compounds. Most of the women who work seasonally are day labourers from the local villages. About half the men are also locals and live close enough to return home every night. In the compounds, however, the ratio of men to women is about seven men to every woman. Since the early 1990s, most of the labourers living in the compounds have come from the adjacent river valley, where overcrowding, severe soil erosion, and persistent drought make migration the main survival strategy for the area's residents. The men are generally not accompanied by either wives or girlfriends.

In the mid-1990s, researchers interested in health promotion conducted a socioeconomic survey on the farm. They have maintained contact since then, and planned to conduct a follow-up random survey 10 years later. The details and objectives were presented to the farm's management in meetings held in their town and farm offices, as well as in written correspondence. Once the management provided consent for the study, the researchers held introductory meetings on each of the farm's compounds to explain their interest in health promotion and the work they would be doing on the farm. The researchers were careful to define their role, stating clearly that they were not advocates for workers' problems. They encouraged the workers to continue to voice any complaints through their own lines of communication with management. They explained that it was in the farm's interest to have healthy workers and they would pass on information to the company about health issues. At these meetings, male workers living in the compounds talked mainly about the large number of men and their need for women, and second about their anxieties and queries about sexually transmitted infections, including HIV/AIDS.

After the introductory meetings, the researchers mapped and observed the physical and social landscape of the farm. Of particular interest was the contact that migrant farm workers had with local residents, the local bar, the nearby border post, prostitutes, their own home areas, and both informal and formal treatment sources. The findings from these exercises highlighted not only the disproportionate number of men to women in two of the three farm compounds, and the fact that most men were unaccompanied by wives or girlfriends, but also that there was sexual contact between some local women and migrant men. This contact usually took place during the early afternoon or weekends, and generally outdoors, hidden from view.

In order to conduct the survey, which was the next stage of the research study, the researchers registered all farm workers, revealing that about 8% of the total workforce was younger than 16 years. Of this subgroup, 68% were local females, aged 8 to 15 years, who worked on the farm on a seasonal basis and lived in the surrounding villages. The researchers were concerned that these young local girls, through their daily contact with migrant men, might be entering into sexual relations, which could expose them to sexually transmitted infections, including HIV. They were also concerned that some of the school-aged workers, especially young girls, chose to continue working instead of returning to school.

Although they recognized the need for people to raise money, the researchers felt that the situation was both wrong and dangerous for the young girls, and could not decide on the most appropriate course of action in response to their observations and early findings.

Questions

1. Should the researchers inform farm management of their findings (that many underage girls are working on the farm) and their concerns (that these underage girls are probably being exposed to sexually transmitted infections, including HIV)?

2. Are the researchers under any ethical obligation to take study participants out of "harm's way" even if they haven't contributed to the risk?

3. If parents knew of the risks to their young daughters and still gave their approval for the work, would it make any difference to what the researcher should do?

4. What obligations do you see as part of the researchers' obligations and which ones are not obligations but are morally justifiable?

Case 55

Interviewing child domestic helpers in sub-Saharan Africa

Child fosterage – the practice in which children leave their birth families to live with other members of their extended kinship or community – is a long-established practice in sub-Saharan Africa. Traditionally, child fosterage involves a reciprocal relationship, with the child providing domestic help in return for care, assistance, and familial affection. Increasingly, however, agents are using the guise of traditional fosterage to recruit girl children and then to traffic them into domestic labour. Instead of receiving the promised care and assistance, these children are vulnerable to exploitation and abuse, which can result in their health being seriously compromised by pregnancies, unsafe abortions, and sexually transmitted infections, including HIV.

Two scientists have designed a questionnaire-based study to identify the type and extent of problems and challenges related to reproductive health among girls age 13-17 years who live outside of their family home and do domestic labour. They also want to determine whether certain factors (such as the socioeconomic background and demographics of the girls, the dominant recruitment method – whether traditional fosterage or trafficking – the type of work they are expected to do as labourers, the kinship relationship with "employers", and the accessibility of community resources) place some domestic workers at greater risk than others. The questionnaires have a mix of questions, and are necessarily personal and probing.

The scientists have chosen four urban sites and, using statistical techniques, have determined the number of interviews they need to conduct to gather useful information. Their strategy for recruiting participants is to have trained interviewers approach dwellings to ask if they have a house helper who is aged younger than 17 years or a foster child who helps with domestic chores. If the response is positive, they will explain that they are doing a study on the health needs of fostered children and would like to ask permission to allow their house helper to participate. If the answer is yes, then they will ask the child for signed informed consent. In order to ensure that the "employer" does not guess the true objective of the study, and to minimize risk to the children including the risk of harassment or a beating, the children will be interviewed in private. Each interviewer will have a separate "safe" questionnaire to revert to should the child's "employer" enter the room unexpectedly, and the child will have been prepared for this possibility. The interviewers will give the children their contact details and information about how to contact a psychologist who is working on the study with them. Both the employers and the house helpers will be given a small amount of money to compensate for time lost due to the interview.

Questions

1 Have the interviewers adequately met their obligation to ensure the interviewees' privacy and confidentiality?

2 Have the interviewers taken adequate precautions to ensure the safety of the interviewees? What other potential risks should they be sensitive to in designing these measures?

3 Who is the appropriate person to give consent in this study and why? Should the consent of a minor be considered valid?

4 Could this study have been done with former child house helpers who might or might not have continued to work in the homes, and still be valid? If the scientists interviewed adult house helpers, would they need to use the same precautions as with the children?

Chapter VIII

Professional Ethics

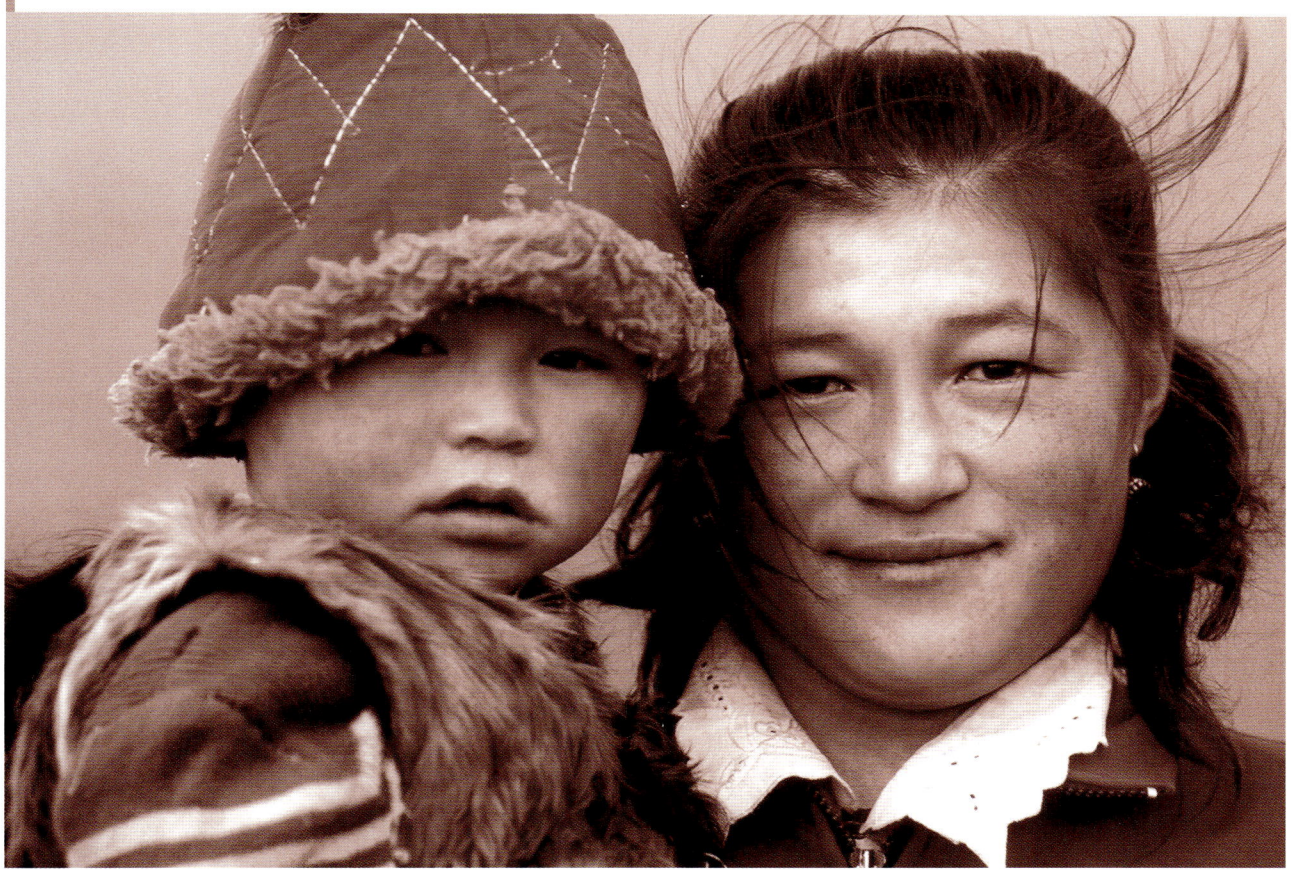

© WHO

Introduction: Chapter VIII

What to do when loyalties are divided?
How should research misbehaviour be defined and policed?

The expectation that researchers and other stakeholders in the research process – including ethics committee members, sponsors, and funders – will act with integrity and honesty is a fair one. When a research article is published, it is fair to expect, at the very least, that the data has not been fabricated, falsified, or plagiarized; that results are correctly reported; that the disclaimers about conflicts of interest are complete and correct; that a thorough and impartial ethical review of the protocol took place before the study began; and that authorship is properly attributed to those who contributed their work. If any of these expectations are not met, the integrity of the research could be called into question, along with the ability and interest of regulatory and professional bodies to govern research activities with the necessary rigour.

Professional ethics covers a broad spectrum of activities and expectations for moral and appropriate behaviour, ranging from expectations about published work, to the professional-conduct issues of abuse, harassment, and intimidation of colleagues or research participants. Whereas some behaviour is clearly wrong and insupportable, other behaviour might be more difficult to clearly identify as such. At what point, for example, does funding from a pharmaceutical company bias or compromise scientific judgment? This chapter draws attention to two broad areas of professional ethics: conflicts of interest and scientific misconduct. The case studies raise the additional issues of abuse of positions of power for personal benefit and regulation of professional ethics.

Conflicts of interest: recognizing and resolving divided loyalites

Conflicts of interest are a relatively new addition to the group of ethical issues that receive widespread attention in the context of international health research. Although conflicts of interest are a familiar concept in the regulation of legal or business relationships that are based on trust, their application to medicine, and in particular to health research, is not yet well conceptualized. Sharp differences of opinion exist both in the specialized literature and among scientists and ethicists over what counts as a conflict of interest and in what circumstances a conflict should be regarded as an ethical problem.

Conflicts of interest as personal gains that can compromise integrity

In the research context, scientists have a conflict of interest if they stand to achieve personal gain (money or the equivalent) by failing to discharge professional obligations either to protect the welfare of participants or to uphold the integrity of the scientific process. An editor of a journal who supplements his income by consulting for a drug company, for example, might accept a submitted manuscript that reported results favourable to that company, not on the basis of its scientific worth, but because not to do so could jeopardize this extra source of income. A growing body of evidence shows that reports of industry-sponsored research are much more likely to be favourable to the sponsor, and that an author who has financial links to a firm is likely to write papers that support that firm's interests. Companies might simply choose to support scientists who favour their products, but certainly the question of conflict arises in this type of case.

It is important to note that the activities that present a potential conflict of interest need not involve any wrongdoing. A lawyer for two legitimate clients might have to withdraw from one or both relationships if one sues the other. The wrong, if any, would consist in failing to do so once the conflict presented itself. Similarly, neither editing a journal nor consulting for a drug company is wrong in itself, but to hold the two roles simultaneously could potentially distort editorial judgment.

Vague as this formulation is, it is useful because it excludes several types of conflict. In particular, it omits the potential tension between patient care and good science, the management of which can be seen as the central rationale for, and responsibility of, the research ethics committee. That conflict is certainly real and important, but it is addressed separately in Chapter I. For clarity, we refer to that type of conflict as a conflict of mission, and reserve the phrase conflicts of interest for cases of personal gain.

Two developments have caused conflicts of interest to become a significant issue in health research involving human beings. First, the rise of private-sector biotechnology companies has vastly expanded the size and scope of industry-funded research, including clinical trials, and thus created many opportunities for financial incentives and gains on the part of clinicians and scientists. Second, increasing numbers of scientists in both developed and developing countries have financial relationships, including equity ownership, with companies that develop and market their discoveries. These changes have transformed the socioeconomic landscape of the life sciences, and particularly of health research. In most medical specialties, appointment of a committee of leading scientists (for example, to review a project) who are totally free from conflicts of interest is nearly impossible, and journals find it difficult to insist that experts who are called upon to review manuscripts or to write survey articles or editorials be free of all financial ties to industry. In countries that have very few experts on whom to call, the situation is likely to be even more complex.

RECs and conflicts of interest

The growth of commercial research ethics committees in industrialized countries, and the introduction of user fees by RECs in developing countries, have fuelled further concerns about potential conflicts of interest. Among some of the perceived advantages of commercial RECs are their capacity to review a high volume of research studies and their ability to provide reviews quickly. The CIOMS *International Ethical Guidelines for Biomedical Research Involving Human Subjects* do not prohibit financial payments to RECs, but state under Guideline 2 that "The review committees must be independent of the research team, and any direct financial or other material benefit they may derive from the research should not be contingent on the outcome of their review."[1] However, to determine or even demonstrate whether financial benefit will undermine the objectivity and independence of the REC is difficult. Some researchers argue that for-profit RECs do not necessarily involve direct financial transactions between research sponsors and reviewers, since reviewers are paid for their work just as the members of RECs for some academic and governmental non-profit organizations are paid in recognition of their time and expertise. Obviously, receiving remuneration for reviewing cannot be considered an unethical practice, although it might become unethical if the remuneration became an incentive, or were found to be consistently linked to the committee providing favourable opinions.

Conflicts of interest can also occur in communities in which research is planned. Community leaders might stand to gain from research in intangible ways, such as enhanced reputation or increased prominence in the community, and might end up trying to please the investigator to the extent that community interests could be given less weight than so-called efficiencies in research. Such conflicts of interest are often difficult for investigators and RECs to detect: investigators might have an implicit complicity in the research project, and RECs often rely on community leaders to speak for their communities.

---

[1] Council for International Organizations of Medical Sciences (CIOMS). International Ethical *Guidelines for Biomedical Research Involving Human Subjects*. Geneva, Switzerland: Council for International Organizations of Medical Sciences (CIOMS) 2002. http://www.cioms.ch/frame_guidelines_nov_2002.htm (accessed 10 April 2008)

Responding to conflicts of interest

There is no consensus on whether these conflicts of interest represent an actual (as opposed to a potential) ethical problem, and, if so, what solutions might be acceptable. The most common response to perceived conflicts of interest is disclosure – for example, authors and peer reviewers must disclose conflicts to journal editors, who publish details of these conflicts so that readers can judge how they could have affected the research. Similarly, research ethics committees might require scientists to disclose conflicts of interest to the committee, and also to prospective participants. However, the effects of this requirement for disclosure are not yet clear. RECs that require disclosure sometimes lack policies that determine which (if any) conflicts are unacceptable, or what action to take if conflicts could potentially compromise the validity of the research. Prospective research participants might not have enough familiarity with research to know how conflicts of interest might affect their interests. Those who rely on research participation to obtain needed health care might have no alternative but to consent, irrespective of whether a disclosure revealed that, for example, a researcher was not only a care provider, but also had a vested interest in the development of a drug being tested. As science and the market continue to become integrated, the need to develop an evidence-based, coherent policy on conflicts of interest will become evident.

REC members might also have conflicts of interest; for example if they have personal or professional links to an investigator whose protocol is being discussed, or if they have financial interests in a company that is sponsoring a trial. If so, they might be reluctant to speak up against the trial design or for enhanced participant protection. RECs therefore need to have policies that require disclosure from their members, and that specify what action should be taken in case of a disclosure (e.g. the member might be asked to leave the room during voting or might not be part of certain discussions). The primary interest of research ethics committees must be the safety and protection of research participants. Secondary interests might include financial gain or recognition. One way to manage the concern that these secondary interests could override the primary interest could be through regulation and monitoring – RECs must develop policies and protocols to address these issues.

Scientific misconduct: Defining and controlling misbehaviour in research

Scientific misconduct in health research – what the Wellcome Trust has described as "the fabrication, falsification, plagiarism or deception in proposing, carrying out or reporting results of research or deliberate, dangerous or negligent deviations from accepted practices in carrying out research"[1] – can undermine the potential of health research to add to human knowledge and to improve the well-being of future patients. Therefore, scientific misconduct must be considered if it is relevant to the ethical evaluation of proposed research.

Like fraud and crime, scientific misconduct is usually hidden by those who perpetrate it, so it is impossible to know how frequently it occurs. In one widely reported survey of scientists in the USA,[2,3] less than 2% admitted to falsifying data, plagiarism or ignoring major aspects of rules and significantly larger numbers admitted to circumventing what they judged to be minor requirements and admitting they had overlooked others' use of flawed data or questionable interpretations. Although data are not available for most other countries, the history of research – including the highly competitive field of health research – reveals numerous scandals involving fraud and deviations from accepted methods.

---

[1] Wellcome Trust. *Statement on the Handling of Allegations of Research Misconduct*. London, UK: Wellcome Trust, 2005. (http://www.wellcome.ac.uk/About-us/Policy/Policy-and-position-statements/WTD002756.htm, accessed 16 June 2008.)

[2] Martinson BC, Anderson MS, DeVries RG. Scientists Behaving Badly. *Nature,* 2005. 435: 737-738. (doi:10.1038/435737a accessed 12 October 2008).

[3] De Vries R, Anderson MS, Martinson BC. Normal Misbehavior: Scientists Talk About the Ethics of Research. *Journal of Empirical Research on Human Research Ethics,* 2006. 1: 43-50.

These practices do not need debating, for they have no defenders. Instead, ethical dilemmas arise when deciding how to respond to misconduct. To whom does the responsibility fall to investigate allegations, to demand and evaluate evidence, and to press for retractions and sanctions? Who, if anyone, should be faulted for failing to take such actions? Who should protect the accused scientist from the harm caused by accusations that are unsupported by evidence? Who must ensure that those who "blow the whistle" do not suffer reprisals, and how?

Whether the definition of misconduct varies among cultures is unclear. What matters is not whether more scientists in one country are dishonest than in another, but whether the same practices are regarded as instances of misconduct regardless of where they occur. A related question is whether certain practices ought to be viewed the same way by everyone, even if culturally distinct views have existed in the past. For example, scientists in one country might underestimate the potential effect of a particular laboratory practice on the production of valid data compared with scientists in another country; irrespective of how consistently these views may have been held in the past, they could simply be normatively mistaken.

If the core issues of research misconduct involve the falsification or misreporting of data, the term is also used to describe a variety of undesirable activities by scientists, such as stealing credit for results, disparaging competitors, or offering a poor role model for students. Although some of these vices can be understood as elements of a distinctive ethic of science,[1] the boundary between these and ordinary aspects of personal character is indistinct.

Many instances of scientific misconduct which occur can be identified with a competent scientific and ethical review, and institutions should have independent guidelines and mechanisms to consider and sanction such issues as scientific and personal integrity and code of conduct, and publication and authorship policies. Journal editors are also responsible for vigilance against possible fraud and misconduct. Many of the issues related to scientific misconduct actually fall under the purview of publication ethics. Not all RECs regard minimizing scientific misconduct as part of their core mandate; many are underfunded and overworked, and have little or no incentive to monitor the conduct of trials after they have been approved. Still, RECs can decrease the possibility of scientific misconduct by setting certain requirements:

1. A competent technical review to examine the justification of a trial, the trial design, and the methods of data analysis.

2. A trial protocol that includes sections on trial monitoring and auditing, data management, and quality assurance.

3. Monitoring of trials if possible, by an independent data safety monitoring board, with regular follow-up, including monitoring visits by the REC to assess the validity of data collection.

4. Registration of research in publicly accessible registers.

5. The raw data from clinical trials should be made available to independent bodies after publication of results to enable verification of the data analysis.

---

[1] Koertge N, ed. *Scientific Values and Civic Virtues*. Oxford, UK: Oxford University Press, 2005.

Suggested readings

Bodenheimer T. Conflict of Interest in Clinical Drug Trials: A Risk Factor for Scientific Misconduct. (2000)

"In clinical drug trials, conflict of interest usually refers to the situation in which an investigator has a financial relationship (often research funding) with a company whose product the investigator is studying. There is nothing intrinsically wrong with conflicts of interest; they are virtually ubiquitous in clinical drug trials because so many trials are funded by the manufacturer of the product being studied. The problem is less conflict of interest itself; the problem is that conflict of interest may be a risk factor for scientific misconduct."

http://www.hhs.gov/ohrp/coi/bodenheimer.htm
(accessed 9 May 2008)

Campbell EG, et al. Financial Relationships Between Institutional Review Board Member and Industry. *New England Journal of Medicine*, 2006; 355(22): 2321-2329.

"Little is known about the nature, extent, and consequences of financial relationships between industry and institutional review board (IRB) members in academic institutions. [The authors] surveyed IRB members about such relationships and [conclude that] relationships between IRB members and industry are common, and members sometimes participate in decisions about protocols sponsored by companies with which they have a financial relationship. Current regulations and policies should be examined to be sure that there is an appropriate way to handle conflicts of interest stemming from relationships with industry."

http://content.nejm.org/cgi/content/full/355/22/2321
(accessed 10 May 2008)

Faunce TA, Jeffrys S. Whistleblowing and Scientific Misconduct: Renewing Legal and Virtue Ethics Foundations. *Medicine and Law*, 2007;26(3):567-584.

"Whistleblowing in relation to scientific research misconduct, despite the benefits of increased transparency and accountability it often has brought to society and the discipline of science itself, remains generally regarded as a pariah activity by many of the most influential relevant organizations. The motivations of whistleblowers and those supporting them continued to be questioned and their actions criticised by colleagues and management, despite statutory protections for reasonable disclosures appropriately made in good faith and for the public interest."

http://www.ncbi.nlm.nih.gov/pubmed/17970253
abstract only (accessed 10 May 2008).

Momen H, Gollogly L. Cross-cultural Perspectives of Scientific Misconduct. *Medicine and Law*, 2007;26(3):409-416.

"The increasing globalization of scientific research lends urgency to the need for international agreement on the concepts of scientific misconduct. Universal spiritual and moral principles on which ethical standards are generally based indicate that it is possible to reach international agreement on the ethical principles underlying good scientific practice […] Defining scientific misconduct to be universally recognized and universally sanctioned means addressing the broader question of ensuring that research is not only well-designed – and addresses a real need for better evidence – but that it is ethically conducted in different cultures."

http://www.ncbi.nlm.nih.gov/pubmed/17970242
abstract only (accessed 10 May 2008)

Case 56

Testing delivery methods for a hormonal contraceptive

The manufacturer of a new hormonal contraceptive commissions a research team to design a clinical trial to compare the effectiveness and tolerability of the new preparation using three different methods of delivery – oral tablets, transdermal patches, and injections. The manufacturer also wants the researchers to focus on the use of this new contraceptive in women of two different socioeconomic groups. The working hypothesis is that the delivery of hormonal contraceptives by transdermal patches or as an injectable depot is as effective and safe as the use of tablets, irrespective of whether or not the users have received secondary education.

The manufacturer draws up a contract with the regional health authorities, which stipulates that the manufacturer will pay the salary of each researcher employed by the regional authorities for the study. The manufacturer further provides each researcher with a personal computer to aid in data collection and storage and pays the researchers an agreed sum of money (about US$ 1000) for each volunteer who completes the trial. The researchers then begin to identify an equal number of suitable participants for the study from each of the two socioeconomic groups. Once the two participant groups are formed, they are randomized to the three modes of delivery of the new contraceptive. The participants are told to discontinue their current contraceptive regimen for the duration of the trial.

Each research participant has the benefit of individual attention during the trial and is provided with the new contraceptive free of charge. The manufacturer pays each volunteer a small amount (about US$ 20) as compensation for possible failure or undesirable side-effects of the new preparation.

Questions

1. All stakeholders in this study receive some benefits. Comment on the appropriateness of each and discuss other types of compensations that could be provided. Are there any conflicts of interest?

2. Are these benefits commensurate with the possible risks?

3. Should partners be involved in the consent process?

4. If the contraceptive technique used before the trial was the condom, what should be done if the woman contracts a sexually transmitted infection, which might include HIV, during the trial?

5. What obligation does the sponsor have towards the research participants if the preparation either fails or has undesirable effects?

Adapted from workshop material developed by the UNDP/UNFPA/WHO/World Bank Special Programme of Research, Development and Research Training in Human Reproduction in Bangkok, Thailand, 2004.

Case 57

Testing a treatment for schizophrenia

An Asian pharmaceutical company has developed a promising new antipsychotic medication for the treatment of schizophrenia.[1] Sales analysts predict the drug could earn the company a substantial profit within four years. The study drug has already been tested on several thousand volunteers in Asia. During this testing, however, some study participants developed cardiac arrhythmias. Consequently, the regulatory agency responsible issued a "not approvable" letter, which requires the drug company to do more tests of the drug on human beings before it can be considered for approval again.

In response, the company contracts a state hospital in eastern Europe to complete the needed tests. The hospital is a long-term facility for mentally ill patients; it is overcrowded, and most patients have been in the facility for many years with no hope of being discharged. Often they have to wait for several months before they get an opportunity to see a doctor. Many patients do not have any next of kin or relatives who visit them regularly or at all.

Facility doctors determine whether a patient is competent to enter a study before obtaining informed consent for their participation. They are paid a small fee for each patient who is recruited. The information sheet given to patients states that the drug "has been tested in thousands of patients and the results of these studies are being reviewed by authorities in Asia, Europe, and the United States of America". It also notes that the drug "appeared to slightly affect the electrical activity of the heart in some people". The company did not inform the eastern European regulators of the Asian regulatory agency's action; the laws of this country do not require such reporting and thus the company contends that it "adheres to the laws of each country in which research is conducted".

Questions

1. Discuss the risk-benefit analysis of this project. Should pharmaceutical companies that apply for drug approval be required to inform other countries of the regulatory agency's concerns, irrespective of the laws of those countries, when testing or marketing the relevant drugs?

2. What are the ethical issues raised by this study?

3. How can competency to give consent best be assured when recruiting mentally ill patients in a busy state institution?

4. Do you think that this study falls in the category of scientific misconduct? Why or why not?

5. Are the doctors who recruit participants for the study in a position of conflict of interest?

6. If the drug works, what, if any, is the obligation of the company to provide it to participants after the trial?

---

[1] A mental disorder characterized by profound disruptions in thinking, affecting language, perception, and the sense of self. It often includes psychotic experiences, such as hearing voices or delusions. It can impair functioning through the loss of an acquired capability to earn a livelihood, or the disruption of studies. Schizophrenia typically begins in late adolescence or early adulthood. Most cases of schizophrenia can be treated, and people affected by it can lead productive lives and be integrated in society.

Case 58

Budget reviews by research ethics committees

A major North American university has submitted a research proposal to the research ethics committee of the National University School of Medicine (NUSM) in a developing country in South-East Asia. It is an ambitious proposal that carries with it a US$ 500 000 yearly budget to examine the efficacy of an innovative national family planning programme The proposal includes bringing researchers to North America for short-term training on new family planning strategies, low-cost surgeries, and programme management. The NUSM research ethics committee has asked the North American university to submit the project budget for the board to consider as part of their evaluation of the entire proposal. The North American university responded that it would prefer the budget review process to be separate from the examination of the scientific and ethical aspects of the proposal. NUSM has a policy of taking 10% of the budget of any collaborative project for overhead, and the North American university is concerned that the size of the budget might unduly sway the committee's decision, especially since so many of the members of both the proposed research group and the ethics committee are from NUSM.

The NUSM REC responds that they will not even consider the proposal if they are not given the budget to review. Their reasoning is as follows:

- They do not want to approve projects that would not have sufficient funding, and North American universities are often out of touch with the realities of the costs of conducting research in their country.

- Budget review is considered a critical piece of their review, as it is only by examining the budget that they can evaluate which institutions will staff various roles, how much money is available for local infrastructure building, and ultimately how much will be given back to the host institution where the research is being conducted.

Questions

1. Is review of a budget within the purview of a research ethics committee? Why, or why not?

2. Is there a potential for conflict of interest in this situation? If so, how might it be addressed?

3. Should a research ethics committee weigh the capacity-building merits of a research proposal (e.g. training, new labs, new building, or computer capability) with the relevance of the research to the country's health problems? If so how?

Adapted from: "Budget Reviews", a case study contributed by Andrea Ruff and Joan Atkinson, Johns Hopkins Bloomberg School of Public Health and Johns Hopkins Berman Institute of Bioethics.

Case 59

Determining the workforce costs of the AIDS epidemic

The staff-benefits group of a west African mining company asks a research team based at a European university to help determine the economic impact of the AIDS epidemic on their workforce. The group wants to convince senior management that the cost is much higher than expected. They suspect that absenteeism due to AIDS, rapid turnover of highly trained and semi-skilled staff (which generates retraining costs), treatment costs associated with the illness, and one-time benefits and funeral costs that must be provided to families of affected workers have been underestimated.

The staff-benefits group hopes that if they demonstrate the costs of the epidemic, the company will focus more attention on preventive programmes. Such programmes could include distribution of pamphlets, holding lectures at the workplace, and organizing recreational activities for single men who live at the company hostels (some of whom frequent a nearby area with a high concentration of commercial sex-workers). Such preventive and educational services could also be provided to the families of married workers. Other interventions might include establishment of clinics to treat sexually transmitted infections more aggressively, or long-term provision of family housing units. The staff-benefits group believes that a report from a well-respected university research group will be an effective way to influence company policy, and promote preventive programmes.

The research team will be fully funded by the company, including overhead payments commensurate with university guidelines. The company has stated that it will not restrict the researchers' ability to publish the study findings, although it will require that the company and all its employees remain anonymous in any reports or publications.

The research centre puts together a team consisting of a physician, an economist, a public health specialist, and a research associate, and travels to the west African country for 3 weeks of intensive fieldwork and investigation. At their request, the team is given access to records of all employees who have had to leave the company because of AIDS or AIDS-related illnesses. Any data that could identify individual employees are removed from the records. No data on the prevalence of infection exist within the company but sample surveys have been done in other parts of the country to examine rates of HIV infection in similar age groups.

As the data-collection phase nears completion and the research team prepares to return home to analyse the data and prepare the report, a senior member of a trade union requests a private meeting with them. He expresses concern that the company will not use the results of the study to improve public health programmes in the company, but will instead conclude that anyone who is HIV-positive will be too costly to the company, and that therefore even HIV-positive individuals who are still healthy will be released on some pretext. Although the company is barred from testing new employees, it can require that employees obtain private health insurance, which often requires an HIV test. Finally, he states that the company will probably cut back its workforce (and therefore decrease its liability) by downsizing and outsourcing.

The team members request a meeting with the sponsors of the research and, without disclosing their source, express their concern that the report could be used for purposes that are contrary to their intentions. The company insists that any rumours they have heard about misuse of the report are untrue. However, the research associate is not satisfied with the company's explanation, and asserts that unless the company provides their assurance in writing, she will immediately withdraw from the project. The company says that it cannot sign such a statement, since doing so would reflect badly on the integrity of the organization.

The research team analyses the data, and presents the following conclusions to the management of the company before publication:

- The prevalence of HIV infection in the general population will probably lead to an employee turnover rate of at least 10% per year for the company.

- Health care costs for the company will increase significantly over the next 5 years and could constitute 15% of its total operational costs. By law, if an employee's illness is diagnosed while working for a company, all health care costs related to that illness must be provided by the company, whether or not the illness is work-related.

- To reduce costs, the company should begin to develop a home-treatment programme for employees with AIDS.

- Prevention programmes will almost certainly reduce the incidence of HIV infection among employees, although the cost-effectiveness of these programmes is not known.

Managers at the company are alarmed by the report and by the projected costs of caring for HIV-positive employees. The CEO says that if the company is forced to take on the health care costs of all employees who become HIV-positive during their employment, the company will be unable to compete in the international market and will be forced to declare bankruptcy or relocate to a lower-cost country that does not make the same health care demands. In either case, everyone at the company will lose their job, leaving many households without any income.

He asks that the research team be sensitive to this issue in writing their conclusions. In fact, he asks the team to recommend that employer-subsidized health insurance plans be allowed to cap benefits for HIV at far less than the costs of the treatment needed. Employees with HIV would then either pay for their own treatment, forgo treatment, or rely on publicly provided services. Households and extended families would probably bear the brunt of the costs, since the health care facilities of the government and non-governmental organizations (NGO) have already been overwhelmed by HIV/AIDS patients. The CEO argues that transferring costs to government, to households, and to other companies is a rational response for a profit-maximizing business. Given the international reputation of the research team, he expresses confidence that government regulators will be influenced to change policies on the basis of a report that recommends a cap on benefits.

Questions

1. Should the research team be concerned about how the data will be used? If so, what provisions could be incorporated to ensure that the report would not be misused?

2. After the report is presented, can the company interpret and use the data any way they so choose?

3. If one or all members of the research team are uncomfortable with the concerns of the CEO, what action could they, or should they, take? If the research team agrees with the CEO, should they include the recommendations that the CEO has suggested?

4. Should the research team have asked the company's executives for their recommendations before sending the results for publication?

Case 60

Action research on involuntary resettlement

A small community-based NGO has been delivering a health programme in the slums of a large city in South Asia. Part of the slum's population has been relocated to another colony, 15 km away, and the NGO has set up a clinic in this new colony. Based on their experience with the community both before and after relocation, the NGO staff members are convinced that the process of resettlement has damaged even further the lives of the people who have been relocated. To expose the living conditions in the new settlement, they set up a partnership with a research organization to study the impact of relocation on the health, education, and livelihoods of the people.

To maintain a distinction between the team of researchers and the local NGO staff, only one person from the NGO assists the research team; their sole responsibilities are to help organize meetings and to conduct sample selection. The researchers hope this will preserve the objectivity of the study and protect the local NGO staff from any negative consequences or backlash from people with vested interests who might resent the study.

Initially, the research team had planned to do several case studies. They propose to choose participants who have been directly affected by the displacement and who seek treatment at the NGO clinic. These people could have experienced discontinuation of treatment, emotional trauma, denial of services at local hospitals, loss of income and buying power, decreased social and family support, or other negative impacts. However, the research ethics committee decides that it would not be ethical to choose participants for case studies from among users of the clinic, since some people might feel that unless they participate in the study, the NGO might not provide health services to them. The committee recommends that the team record any such cases that they encounter during a household survey. Members of the NGO did not agree with this decision, and don't see a problem with doing case studies based on clinic patients. Since patients often visit the clinic, the NGO staff believe that the patients would give more detailed information about their experiences and problems than would randomly selected respondents, many of whom might not even know about either the clinic or the NGO.

Nonetheless, the research team decide to do a household level survey by selecting a systematic random sample. In doing so, the research team realize that the people are frustrated with the amount of checking by the government to verify their claims and identify illegal residents. The research team are able to function only by identifying themselves with the NGO. Although this brings them greater acceptance, it also puts them under pressure to provide direct assistance to the people, such as escorting sick community members to the hospital, counselling emotionally disturbed individuals, and helping children to get admission to school.

As a consequence, the research team is torn between the need to assist the people and the need to complete their data collection and analysis. The blurring of boundaries between the research team and the NGO has also confused study participants. Although the research team members provide an information sheet that explains the research, and uses a thorough process to obtain informed consent from participants, people often give information in the hope of receiving services. When these people realize that participation will not result in any immediate action, they are often upset. At the same time, the NGO staff are getting impatient with the research team for not incorporating their insights and experiences, because they don't fit in with the study design. The NGO feels that the study is not achieving its original aim, which was to produce material to start a campaign.

Questions

1 Was the ethics committee justified in its decision to disallow the use of clinic patients for case studies? What are the pros and cons of such a design?

2 How far should the research team have gone in fulfilling the community's expectations of direct assistance? What kind of provisions should they have made to meet such an exigency?

3 What are the ethical implications of the research team identifying itself with the local organization? Does this association affect the procedure of informed consent?

4 What are the ethical dilemmas posed by the dual and simultaneous needs of action and research in such situations? How can such dilemmas be resolved?

Adapted from "Action Research on Involuntary Settlements", a case study contributed by Neha Madhiwalla, Centre for Studies in Ethics and Rights, Mumbai and Sahayog, Mumbai, India

Case 61

Victimizing the system or a victim of it?

Xue Lee, a 25-year-old research assistant with plans to go to medical school, has discovered that a set of data given to her by a much-admired senior researcher, Dr Simpson, does not support the working hypothesis of their lab, which is that the increased vulnerability to cardiovascular disease that accompanies ageing is due to changes in the ratio of different levels of lipids or fats in the blood.

Ms Lee shows the unexpected results to Dr Simpson, who takes the file home with him to review. The following week, Dr Simpson returns the database to her with a request that she re-run the statistical analysis now that some mistaken entries had been corrected. Analysis of the new data set gives results that are consistent with the hypothesis of the study. However, Ms Lee notices that all the numbers that were inconsistent with the hypothesis have been changed. When she asks Dr Simpson about this, he dismisses her concerns as unimportant.

Ms Lee shares her misgivings about Dr Simpson's actions with a handful of graduate students and discovers that others have also seen suspicious behaviour from him. She then approaches Dr Jacobs, a faculty member who has collaborated with Dr Simpson in the past. Dr Jacobs advises her that no matter how she proceeds, everyone will lose; if she could prove that he has altered the data, Ms Lee's own reputation would probably suffer. Dr Jacobs cautions her that whatever her course of action, she should be sure that she has iron-clad evidence. This would especially be necessary in light of the fact that Dr Simpson has been recruited to the university because of his reputation as a person who can win grants; he has succeeded in securing US$ 3 million for the university in his first year.

Ms Lee continues to review other data sets and begins to see a pattern of data manipulation, including reversing data points, figures for measurements that have never been done, and data from patients who do not exist. She becomes convinced that she is seeing not just a few lapses in ethical judgement, but calculated scientific fraud. She lodges a formal, written accusation of scientific misconduct against her former mentor 3 months after she first discovered the altered numbers. When Dr Simpson is confronted by the department chairman the next day, he denies the accusations and suggests that the errors are due to the high number of technicians and post-docs who have handled the data over several years. Notebooks and other material necessary for an investigation are impounded from Dr Simpson's lab 2 days later.

Five faculty members are picked by the dean of the medical school to mount an inquiry into Dr Simpson's work. The informal examination quickly expands beyond the initial complaint to include a review of Dr Simpson's computer hard drive. Numerous interviews are also conducted. Soon, the initial inquiry progresses to a formal investigation, at which point Dr Simpson begins to claim he is a victim. He accuses Ms Lee of being "out to get him" because of personal differences between them and Ms Lee's disapproval of his lifestyle. Dr Simpson's defense slowly unravels, however, and within 2 years he pleads guilty to falsifying information on a federal grant application and agrees to pay the university (and Ms Lee's lawyer) almost US$ 200 000.

The evidence clearly suggests that Dr Simpson has been committing fraud for more than 10 years. Although he has taken responsibility for his actions, when he appears in federal court for sentencing, he pleads with the court for leniency and a reduced sentence on the following grounds:

- The pressure of his academic position caused him to use poor judgement, since he felt that he would be evaluated primarily by the number of grants (and money) that he brought to the university;

- He felt responsible for all the people in his lab, especially the doctoral students and post-docs who depended on him for funding;

- He did not want the money for himself but to support others and their research; and

- Being awarded the grants gave him a sense of self-worth and prestige, which had motivated him to do community service in teaching science to primary-school children. He expresses his intention to continue this service if the court suspends his sentence.

Questions

1 Do you think that Dr Simpson has given valid reasons to account for his falsifying the data in his studies?

2 Whistle blowing is not always seen in a positive manner. Should Ms Lee be rewarded – or disciplined – for bringing this case to light and, if so, in what way?

3 What, if any, is the role of a research ethics committee in this situation? Whose responsibility is it to enforce scientific integrity?

Case 62

Truth and consequences

Six graduate students who work under Professor Maria Kieros in the department of genetics at a major university have reluctantly come to the conclusion that she has been faking data. This conclusion is based on a number of direct and indirect observations. In reading a grant application, for example, Ms Heath, one of the graduate students, has noted that some data was represented as if it were unpublished data even though it had appeared in an earlier paper published by the laboratory. Other graduate students have noted that certain data seemed to have been manipulated. On the advice of two university scientists, the group confronts Prof Kieros with their observations. She is very defensive and blames the problem on a computer error. Some of the students are convinced by this explanation; others worry that other grant applications including two that have been funded, could be fraudulent. Moreover, Ms Heath and others are growing concerned about progress with their own studies. Despite months of work, Ms Heath has been unable to replicate observations that were reported by Prof Kieros in earlier papers.

The mounting unease among the students makes it necessary for them to decide as a group whether or not to make their observations public. Alerting the administration creates the possibility that their own research will be called into question. If Prof Kieros is found guilty, they will probably have to restart their research efforts, adding years to their doctoral work. Given the potential for such significant consequences, the students agree not to approach the university administration unless the desire to do so is unanimous.

Almost 7 months after members of the group first suspect fraud in Prof Kieros' data, the group finally takes the matter to two university deans. The deans initiate an informal inquiry during which they find evidence that leads them to endorse a formal investigation into Prof Kieros' work a few weeks later. News that Prof Kieros' students have made the charges begins to circulate among other faculty members, along with rumours suggesting that she has had to fake data because her students are not productive enough.

Prof Kieros resigns 2 months later, and after 3 months the university releases its report, which concludes that there is clear evidence of falsification of data in the applications for the cancelled grants. Questions are also raised about three published papers (none of which were co-authored by the graduate students). Lastly, the investigative team notes that Prof Kieros has behaved unprofessionally towards some of her graduate students by pressuring them to conceal research results that disagreed with desired outcomes and urging them to over-interpret data to fit with her hypothesis.

When several of the graduate students meet their thesis committees, their prospects are poor. Prof Kieros' relentless optimism about the lab's work has led some of the students to follow false leads. One of the six students is permitted to continue with her project; two students are told that their work is unusable and they will have to start again with new doctoral projects; three students leave the university. For those who continue with their studies, their graduation is delayed by at least 3 years. As one graduate student says, "We unintentionally suffered the consequences of trying to do the right thing".

Questions

1. Given the consequences to their own work, should the students have reported their concerns about Prof Kieros?

2. What might have happened if they had said nothing and just tried to get through the process so they could graduate?

3. What responsibilities did the university have to the students? How could the university have protected the students from the consequences of their action?

4. How should universities, in general, treat those who are "whistle-blowers"?

Case 63

The curious career of Dr Taylor

For almost three decades, Dr Taylor had a prosperous career at a well-respected North American university, during which he became a world-renowned expert in the fields of nutrition and immunology. He was often nominated for, and had received, prestigious awards and recognitions.

While at the university, Dr Taylor was asked by a company based in the United States of America, Blake Pharmaceuticals, to undertake a large study to test whether their new infant formula could help babies avoid allergies. The study was conducted under the direction of Dr Mason, a clinical research associate at the company. Ms Hughes, Dr Taylor's research nurse, was in charge of finding 288 newborns with allergy-prone parents who were willing to take part in the study. This task was difficult because the city was not only small but was also located in a region with a low birth rate. The prevalence of asthma was relatively low, and at least half the newborns were breastfed. Around the same time, a large European food company, Nutristar, hired Dr Taylor to scientifically test their new infant formula, which they claimed could help to reduce the risk to infants of developing asthma.

By the following summer, no data had been collected for the Blake Pharmaceuticals study, since Ms Hughes had only been able to recruit a quarter of the participants that were needed. Ms Hughes was therefore shocked to discover that the results of the Nutristar study had already been published. The publication also caught the attention of Dr Mason, who was further surprised to see that the study compared the Nutristar and Blake formulas, despite no request for Blake to provide the thousands of clinically labelled cans of their formula that would be required for such a study. Dr Mason confronted Dr Taylor about the Nutristar study, even asking who had labelled all the formula cans used in the study if it had not been done by Blake. Dr Taylor claimed that his team had labelled the cans at the university lab, a claim which Dr Mason found suspicious, since feeding the infants enrolled in the study would have required 20 000 cans of formula.

Shortly after the Nutristar publication, Dr Taylor published yet another infant formula study, for a third company. This study had enrolled more than 200 babies. Taken together, Dr Taylor's three studies would have involved more than 700 babies. Ms Hughes, however, had not seen any of these infants and was convinced that the purported participants in Dr Taylor's studies did not exist, and that it would not have been possible for him to do a study of such magnitude without her knowledge. Her suspicion that Dr Taylor was committing fraud was solidified when she happened to find a paper he was preparing for publication – a 5-year follow-up on the Nutristar study, which she was certain had never been conducted. Hughes decided to report Dr Taylor to the university.

The university assembled an independent panel to investigate the allegations. Members of the panel spent 3 months interviewing witnesses and examining five of Dr Taylor's publications but never made their findings public. They claimed they could not do so because they had signed a confidentiality agreement. The media, however, obtained a copy of the report with its conclusions that the baby formula studies had never been done and that Dr Taylor was guilty of scientific misconduct. Despite these allegations, the university decided not to take any action against Dr Taylor. It later emerged that Dr Taylor had accused the committee of bias, and had threatened to sue. As a publicly funded institution, the administration was concerned that a lawsuit would be costly to the university, and would tarnish its reputation and cause a loss of future income.

In the meantime, Dr Taylor submitted his 5-year follow-up on the Nutristar study to a paediatric medical journal in another country. The article had remained unpublished during the university investigation, but was published after the journal's editors were informed by the university that there was insufficient evidence against Dr Taylor.

Dr Taylor later submitted a study to a prominent European medical journal on the effects of his own patented multivitamin on the memory of elderly people. His results were so impressive that one of the journal's senior editors was sure something was amiss. He sent the study to two reviewers, both of whom expressed their strong doubts about the authenticity of the study. Further, when Dr Taylor was asked to submit his data, he claimed that it had been lost by the university. Since, the journal requires authors to produce all original data upon request, his reaction led many to assume that the study had been invented.

The journal rejected the study and asked Dr Taylor's university to investigate. Two senior university officials headed the inquiry into Dr Taylor's multivitamin study. While the investigation was pending, Dr Taylor submitted the study to another journal, which published the study later that year. The dramatic improvements Dr Taylor reported were so impressive that his study caught the attention of the popular press, putting the doctor and his research in the spotlight all across the country.

The study intrigued two professors, who looked to the original study data to corroborate the amazing results. Their examination revealed a number of glaring errors in Dr Taylor's work. First, they noted that it would have been impossible for the doctor to test the strength of each vitamin in his patented preparation separately and at different strengths on his own. Such an undertaking would require a tremendous amount of work and extensive resources. Second, if the study participants' scores on the memory tests administered at the outset of the study were accurate, the participants "would have to be in such advanced stages of dementia that they would be unlikely to understand the concept of a research study". However, after 1 year of taking Dr Taylor's multivitamin, the participants' scores on the same tests were reported to be normal, which the professors asserted was "ridiculous". According to the professors, the only possible explanation for the study was that Dr Taylor "made it up".

Despite the controversy surrounding his work, Dr Taylor continued to publish. Less than a year after the article in the popular press appeared, he published a study that supported the findings of his controversial multivitamin research in his own journal, Nutrition Research. Soon after, that journal published a study by a Dr Morallon, substantiating data from a study Dr Taylor had published 10 years earlier, the legitimacy of which had also been questioned. Subsequent attempts to contact Dr Morallon failed; he had no e-mail address and, although his institutional affiliation was in Asia, his mailbox was in the United States of America. No other papers authored by him have been found.

At the end of that academic year, Dr Taylor retired, which he claimed he had always planned to do at that time. Since then, he has travelled the world speaking at conferences, continued to publish studies, and has developed a business around his multivitamin. To date, the only study of his that has been retracted is the Nutristar study, despite the fact that at least ten others have been deemed highly suspicious or outright fraudulent.

Questions

1. Did the university do everything it could to investigate Dr Taylor? Did it have an obligation to inform the scientific community and the journals that were considering Dr Taylor's work about the concerns? For what other reasons might the university have hesitated to discipline Dr Taylor?

2. If, after an inquiry, there are no formal sanctions against Dr Taylor, and he subsequently submits a research protocol to a research ethics committee for approval, can committee members legitimately raise questions or express concerns about his credibility or alleged ethical conduct if the study is otherwise completely acceptable? Would they be justified in blocking the study if they believed that the independent panel had been bullied by Dr Taylor, as was proven to be the case?

3. What role does and should the government have, if any, in addressing scientific fraud? What is and should be the role of professional societies?

4. Do the journals that have published papers that are suspected to be fraudulent have any ethical obligation to review other papers that they have already published?

Case 64

Whose idea is it, anyway?

Dr Ruiz is a very productive physician-scientist at a Central American medical research institute in country A, and has completed more than 15 studies and published more than 20 papers. More than 70% of the protocols he has submitted for funding have been approved and implemented. After 5 years, he returns to his home country (country B, also in Central America), leaving behind several ongoing, unfinished studies in the hands of his co-investigators. He also leaves behind unfunded protocols that he wrote with co-investigators at the medical research institute, a few of which have been submitted to funding agencies and are still awaiting funding decisions.

A year after he left the medical research institute, Dr Ruiz is asked by an international research-funding organization to evaluate a research proposal to determine whether it should be supported. The proposal has been submitted by Dr L Lopez, an internationally known clinical investigator and director of an important research unit in another Central American nation (country C). After reading the first few pages, Dr Ruiz realizes he has seen this proposal before; it is, in fact, almost an exact copy of an unfunded proposal that he had written with co-investigators, although the proposal contains no references to or acknowledgements of the institute or any of his co-investigators.

When he informs the funding agency that the proposal has been copied, the agency decides not to finance the study and asks Dr Ruiz to keep the matter strictly confidential. Dr Ruiz, however, is not content to let the matter rest. He feels that this is an egregious example of plagiarism that raises important questions. Dr Lopez, for example, is widely quoted in the literature and is often called upon to consult for international organizations on matters of child health. Dr Ruiz believes that since Dr Lopez has plagiarized his protocol, he could have plagiarized others, and could even have manipulated data. At his request, the funding agency agrees to investigate the matter.

The funding agency reports that it has convened an internal committee, which has thoroughly investigated the incident, and reviewed an explanation provided by Dr Lopez. The committee has concluded that "although negligence may have occurred in the preparation of the proposal, there was no intention to copy the proprietary text of another researcher" and that "no action should be taken against Dr Lopez in this case". The committee also notes that the proposal was the property of Dr Ruiz's former employer, and was not published or copyrighted by him. The funding agency therefore regards the proposal as being in the public domain and thinks that no law was broken when it was copied by Dr Lopez and his colleagues. Dr Ruiz is thanked for his vigilance but given no further explanation.

Dr Ruiz is stunned both by the process of the investigation and by the committee's decision. Neither he nor his co-investigators have been contacted during the investigation. Nor was any enquiry directed to his former employer to find out how Dr Lopez obtained the original proposal. Dr Ruiz further observes that in his current institution, any researcher caught plagiarizing would be suspended from all ongoing research, removed from all research committees, and not allowed to consult internationally until the matter had been completely resolved.

Questions

1 Do you think the funding agency handled this situation appropriately? Why or why not?

2 Did the funding agency use a different standard with regard to the issue of plagiarism because Dr Ruiz was from a developing country rather than from a developed country?

3 Is it unethical to take credit for authorship of a study if you have not written any of the protocol?

4 To which ethical standards should an investigator be held accountable: the standards of his or her own country or society? The country of the funding agency? An international code?

5 How would you address the following scenario: Dr Lopez wishes to conduct the research since he views it as important for country C. He approaches Dr Ruiz and asks to conduct the study, agreeing to give full credit to Dr Ruiz for his contribution. Dr Ruiz, however, refuses to give permission, saying that he plans to do the research sometime in the future in country B. Can Dr Lopez still undertake the study using the research plan developed by Dr Ruiz? In other words, does Dr Ruiz own the idea? If so, for how long?

6 How would you address the following scenario: one of the proposals on which Dr Ruiz worked when he was at the medical research institute in country A has now been submitted by his co-investigators in their own name to a funding agency in that country. When the agency agrees to fund the project, do the co-investigators have to include Dr Ruiz in the grant and involve him in the research, given that he has left country A, and was not involved in the final submission of the proposal for funding? What if the co-investigators have completed data collection and analysis on one of the studies that was ongoing when Dr Ruiz left the medical research institute? Must Dr Ruiz be involved in the writing and submission of any papers growing out of the study, or is it acceptable to publish the paper without listing him as an author because he was not involved in collecting or analysing the data? If he were given an acknowledgement in the publication, would that be a matter of courteous treatment of a fellow scientist or acknowledgement of his original intellectual contribution to, and hence intellectual ownership of the research design?

Glossary[1]

Action Research: *see* **Research design**

Adjuvant therapy: Treatment that is given in addition to the primary treatment. For example, adjuvant therapy for cancer usually refers to surgery followed by chemotherapy or radiotherapy to help decrease the risk of the cancer coming back.

Adenocarcinoma: a malignant tumor originating in glandular (secretary) tissue.

Adverse event (AE): In the context of a clinical trial, any untoward medical occurrence in a patient or clinical investigation subject administered a pharmaceutical product and which does not necessarily have a causal relationship with this treatment. An adverse event can therefore be any unfavourable and unintended sign (including an abnormal laboratory finding), symptom, or disease temporally associated with the use of a medicinal (investigational) product, whether or not related to the medicinal (investigational) product.

Adverse drug reaction (ADR): In the pre-approval clinical experience with a new medicinal product or its new usages, particularly as the therapeutic dose(s) may not be established: all noxious and unintended responses to a medicinal product related to any dose should be considered adverse drug reactions. The phrase responses to a medicinal product means that a causal relationship between a medicinal product and an adverse event is at least a reasonable possibility, i.e. the relationship cannot be ruled out. Regarding marketed medicinal products, an adverse drug reaction is a response to a drug which is noxious and unintended and which occurs at doses normally used in man for prophylaxis, diagnosis, or therapy of diseases or for modification of physiological function. *See also* **Serious adverse event (SAE)** and **Serious adverse drug reaction (Serious ADR)**.

Alcoholism: generally taken to refer to chronic continual drinking or to periodic consumption of alcohol characterized by impaired control over drinking, frequent episodes of intoxication, preoccupation with alcohol and the use of alcohol despite adverse consequences. The term is not exact and, therefore, the narrower formulation of "alcohol dependence syndrome" as one among a wide range of alcohol-related problems is often used instead and refers to a cluster of behavioural, cognitive, and physiological phenomena that may develop after repeated substance use.

Allopathic: conventional evidence-based medical practice in contrast to homeopathy, ayurveda, and alternative therapies and interventions.

Anaemia: a condition in which the haemoglobin concentration in the blood is below a defined level, resulting in a reduced oxygen-carrying capacity of red blood cells. About half of all cases of anaemia can be attributed to iron deficiency; other common causes include infections, such as malaria and schistosomiasis, and genetic factors. The major health consequences include poor pregnancy outcome, impaired physical and cognitive development, increased risk of morbidity in children, and reduced work productivity in adults. Pregnant women and children are particularly vulnerable. Anaemia contributes to 20% of all maternal deaths.

Antipsychotic drug: a drug used to treat psychosis, a group of mental disorders characterized by confusion, delusions, and hallucinations.

Antiretroviral (ARV): a group of medicines used in the treatment of HIV/AIDS. Antiretroviral treatment (ART) suppresses or stops the HIV retrovirus that causes AIDS.

Anonymous: a record, biological sample or item of information that in no circumstance can be linked to an identified person.[2]

---

[1] Glossary definitions and explanations have primarily come from WHO publications. Where they have not, the source has been cited.

[2] Council for International Organizations of Medical Sciences. *International Ethical Guidelines for Biomedical Research Involving Human Subjects.* http://www.cioms.ch/ (accessed 9 May 2008)

Anonymization: (to make anonymous) Research records or biological samples from which all direct or indirect identifiers have been removed such that no link is possible between the records or samples and the identity of the person who was the source of the record or sample.[1]

Anthropometry: the study of the measurement of the human body in terms of the dimensions of bone, muscle, and adipose (fat) tissue.

Arrhythmia: an irregularity in the force or rhythm of the heartbeat. In some cases it can cause cardiac arrest and sudden death.

Audit: (in the context of clinical trials) a systematic and independent examination of trial-related activities and documents to determine whether the evaluated trial-related activities were conducted, and the data were recorded, analyzed, and accurately reported according to the protocol, sponsor's standard operating procedures, good clinical practice, and the applicable regulatory requirements.[2]

Ayurveda: an ancient system of health care that is native to the Indian subcontinent. The word "Ayurveda" is a derived from the sanskrit words *āyus* meaning "life", "life principle", or "long life" and the word *veda*, which refers to a system of "knowledge". Ayurveda means "the knowledge needed for long life". According to the Ayurveda principles, health or sickness depends on the presence or absence of a balanced state of the total body matrix including the balance between its different constituents. Both the intrinsic and extrinsic factors can cause disturbance in the natural equilibrium giving rise to disease. This loss of equilibrium can happen by dietary indiscrimination, undesirable habits, and non-observance of rules of healthy living. The treatment consists of restoring the balance of disturbed body-mind matrix through regulating diet, correcting life-routine and behaviour, administration of drugs, and resorting to preventive therapy.[3]

Beneficence: the ethical obligation to maximize benefit and to minimize harm. This principle gives rise to norms requiring that the risks of research be reasonable in the light of the expected benefits, that the research design be sound, and that the investigators be competent both to conduct the research and to safeguard the welfare of the research participants. Beneficence further proscribes the deliberate infliction of harm on people; this aspect of beneficence is sometimes expressed as a separate principle, of "non-maleficence" (to do no harm).[4]

Beta-carotene: an antioxidant found in many vegetables which is partly converted to vitamin A by the liver. Scientists believe that beta-carotene as found in fresh fruit and vegetables has properties that can contribute to reducing cancer and heart disease.

Blinding or masking: a procedure in which one or more parties to the trial are kept unaware of the treatment assignments. Single-blinding usually refers to the participants being unaware, and double-blinding usually refers to the participants, investigators, monitors, and, in some cases, data analysts being unaware of the treatment assignments.[5]

Cancer: a generic term for a group of more than 100 diseases that can affect any part of the body. Other terms used are malignant tumours and neoplasms. One defining feature of cancer is the rapid creation of abnormal cells which grow beyond their usual boundaries, and which can invade adjoining parts of the body and spread to other organs, a process referred to as metastasis. Metastases are the major cause of death from cancer. Cancer is a leading cause of death worldwide. From a total of 58 million deaths worldwide in 2005, cancer accounts for 7.6 million (or 13%) of all deaths

---

[1] Council for International Organizations of Medical Sciences. *International Ethical Guidelines for Epidemiological Studies*. http://www.cioms.ch/ (accessed 19 May 2009)

[2] International Conference on Harmonization. Guideline for Good Clinical Practice E6(R1). Current Step 4 version.
http://www.ich.org/cache/compo/276-254-1.html (accessed 9 May 2008)

[3] Ministry of Health and Family Welfare, India. Department of Ayurveda, Yoga & Naturopathy, Unani, Siddha and Homeopathy.
http://indianmedicine.nic.in/ayurveda.asp (accessed 9 May 2008)

[4] Council for International Organizations of Medical Sciences (CIOMS) in collaboration with the World Health Organization (WHO). International Ethical Guidelines for Biomedical Research Involving Human Subjects. Op. cit.

[5] International Conference on Harmonization. Guideline for Good Clinical Practice E6(R1). ICH, 1996. http://www.ich.org/cache/compo/276-254-1.html (accessed 9 May 2008)

***Carcinoma in situ* (CIS):** an early form of carcinoma (malignant cancer). It is an accumulation of neoplastic (abnormal) cells that have not spread to surrounding tissues. If left untreated, *carcinoma in situ* can transform into cancer.

Case-control study: *see **Research design**.*

Chlamydia: a sexually transmitted infection caused by the small bacterium *Chlamydia trachomatis*. More cases of STI are caused by *C trachomatis* than by any other bacterial pathogen, making *C trachomatis* infections an enormous public health problem throughout the world. In both men and women, but more so in men, silent, asymptomatic infection is common. The bacterium is transmitted from one partner to another by sexual intercourse. In men it can cause inflammation of the urethra, conjunctiva, or the joins, and in women, it can cause acute inflammation of the reproductive tract, leading to complications such as infertility, potentially fatal ectopic pregnancy, or chronic pain.

Chloroquine: a drug long used in the treatment or prevention of malaria. Over time, the species of protozan parasite *Plasmodium falciparum* that causes the worst malaria in humans, has developed widespread resistance against chloroquine.

Clinical trial: any research study that prospectively assigns individual research participants, or groups of research participants, to one or more health-related interventions to evaluate the effects on health outcomes. Interventions include but are not restricted to drugs, cells and other biological products, surgical procedures, radiologic procedures, devices, behavioral treatments, process-of-care changes, and preventive care.

Cholera: an acute intestinal infection caused by ingestion of food or water contaminated with the bacterium *Vibrio cholerae*. It has a short incubation period, from less than one day to five days, and produces an enterotoxin, a harmful substance that causes a copious, painless, watery diarrhoea that can quickly lead to severe dehydration and death if treatment is not promptly given. Vomiting also occurs in most patients. Cholera is an easily treatable disease. The prompt administration of oral rehydration salts to replace lost fluids nearly always results in cure. In especially severe cases, intravenous administration of fluids may be required to save the patient's life. Left untreated, however, cholera can kill quickly following the onset of symptoms.

CIOMS International Ethical Guidelines for Biomedical Research Involving Human Subjects: The Council for International Organizations of Medical Sciences (CIOMS) is an international nongovernmental organization in official relations with the World Health Organization (WHO). It was founded under the auspices of WHO and the United Nations Educational, Scientific and Cultural and Organization (UNESCO) in 1949 with among its mandates that of maintaining collaborative relations with the United Nations and its specialized agencies, particularly with UNESCO and WHO. The CIOMS Guidelines, are designed to be of use to countries in defining national policies on the ethics of biomedical research involving human subjects, applying ethical standards in local circumstances, and establishing or improving ethical review mechanisms. A particular aim is to reflect the conditions and the needs of low-resource countries, and the implications for multinational or transnational research in which they may be partners.[1] Like the *Declaration of Helsinki* (see separate entry), the CIOMS Guidelines provide important guidance on the ethical conduct of health research.

CIOMS International Ethical Guidelines for Epidemiological Studies: The Council for International Organizations of Medical Science (CIOMS) Guidelines for Epidemiological Studies provide ethical guidance for epidemiologists, as well as those who sponsor, review, or participate in epidemiological studies, on identifying and responding to the ethical issues that are raised by the process of producing this knowledge.[2]

---

[1] Council for International Organizations of Medical Sciences (CIOMS) in collaboration with the World Health Organization (WHO). International Ethical Guidelines for Biomedical Research Involving Human Subjects. Geneva, Switzerland: CIOMS, 2002.

[2] Council for International Organizations of Medical Sciences (CIOMS) in collaboration with the World Health Organization (WHO). International Ethical Guidelines for Epidemiological Studies. Geneva, Switzerland: CIOMS, 2009. http://www.cioms.ch/frame_ethical_guidelines_2009.htm (accessed 19 May 2009)

Community: can be defined as groups of people who can be identified by a shared place of residence (location or neighbourhood) or activity (e.g. employment), or who identify around an identity, activity, or function.

Confidentiality: the obligation to keep information secret unless its disclosure has been appropriately authorized by the person concerned or, in extraordinary circumstances, by the appropriate authorities.

Data safety monitoring board (DSMB) or committee: Constituted and functioning under the authority of the sponsor, a data safety monitoring board is an independent advisory body responsible for assessing data during the course of a study in a manner that contributes to the scientific and ethical integrity of the study. The board's recommendations provide the sponsor with an overall scientific, safety, and ethical appreciation of the study, and should assist the sponsor in maintaining the rigour of the study design, with appropriate attention paid to the protection of human participants.

Deception research: *see Research design*.

Declaration of Helsinki: This declaration by the World Medical Association (WMA) serves as a statement of ethical principles to provide guidance to physicians and others involved in medical research with human beings and identifiable human material or identifiable data.[1] It is one of the most widely known and accepted guideline documents for research ethics. Amendments and clarifications have been made to the original 1964 Declaration and the WMA stresses that the most recent version (2008) is the only one in effect.

Double-blind study: *see Research design or Blinding/Masking*.

Dysentery: any of various disorders marked by inflammation of the intestines, especially of the colon, and attended by abdominal pain and frequent stools containing blood and mucus. Causes include chemical irritants, bacteria, protozoa, and parasitic worms.

Dysplasia: abnormal development or growth of tissues, organs, or cells. It is the earliest form of precancerous lesion. Dysplasia can be diagnosed as either high or low grade, with high grade dysplasia indicative of a more advanced progression towards malignant transformation.

Electroencephalography (EEG): a painless, non-invasive, and safe procedure whereby the electrical activity of the brain is registered, amplified, and recorded by placing electrodes in a specific manner on the head.

Effectiveness: the degree to which an intervention or treatment has a definite or desired effect in real life.[2]

Efficacy: the extent to which an intervention can have a desired effect under ideal or controlled circumstances, such as in a clinical trial. Efficacy is a subset of effectiveness.

End-point: the point in a trial or other type of research at which the predetermined target or goal has been reached.

Epidemiology: the study of the distribution and determinants of health-related states or events in a specific population, and the application of this study to control of health problems.[3]

---

[1] World Medical Association. Declaration of Helsinki as adopted by the WMA General Assembly, October 2008. This 2008 version replaces the original 1964 versions and all subsequent versions.

[2] Nuffield Council on Bioethics. Public Health: Ethical Issues. London, UK: Nuffield Council on Bioethics, 2007.

[3] Last J. A Dictionary of Epidemiology. 4th edn. Oxford, UK: Oxford University Press, 2001.

Equity: the fair distribution of benefits and burdens. Equity is the absence of avoidable or remediable differences among populations or groups defined socially, economically, demographically, or geographically; thus, health inequities involve more than inequality – whether in health determinants or outcomes, or in access to the resources needed to improve and maintain health – but also a failure to avoid or overcome such inequality that infringes human rights norms or is otherwise unfair. In some circumstances, therefore, an equal distribution of benefits and burdens will be considered fair, whereas in others it might be equitable to give preference to those who are in most need or are the most vulnerable. A characteristic common to groups that experience health inequities (e.g. poor or marginalized people, racial and ethnic minorities, and women) is lack of power in political, social, and/or economic terms. Thus, to be effective and sustainable, interventions that aim to redress inequities must typically go beyond remedying a particular health inequality and also help to empower the group in question through systemic changes, such as law reform, changes in economic or social relationships, or the like.

Ethnicity: the collective identity shared by a group of people of common descent or origin.

Equipoise: a state of genuine uncertainty on the part of the expert medical community about the comparative therapeutic merits of each arm in a trial.

Focus group discussion (FGD): a group discussion between 6-12 people, guided by a facilitator, during which group members talk freely and spontaneously about a certain topic. The purpose of using this qualitative research methodology is to obtain in-depth information on the concepts, perceptions, and ideas of a group. A focus group discussion is not designed to be a way of rapidly conducting multiple interviews, developing consensus, making decisions, or providing an opportunity for questions and answers.[1]

Gender: the socially constructed roles, behaviours, activities, and attributes that a given society considers appropriate for men and women (as opposed to sex, which refers to those which are biologically determined). To put it another way, "male" and "female" are sex categories, whereas "masculine" and "feminine" are gender categories. Aspects of sex do not vary substantially between different human societies, whereas aspects of gender can vary greatly.

Gender discrimination: any distinction, exclusion or restriction made on the basis of socially constructed gender roles and norms which prevents a person from enjoying full human rights.

Gentamycin: an antibiotic used to treat many different bacterial infections. Gentamycin is not effective when given orally because it is deactivated when absorbed by the small intestine and filtered into the liver. It can only be given intravenously, intramuscularly, or topically.

Gonorrhoea: a sexually transmitted infection caused by the bacterium *Neisseria gonorrhoeae*. Although gonorrhoea can often be asymptomatic in both men and women, it is usually characterized by genital discharge, painful urination, inflammation and infection of the urethra, and, in women, inflammation of the reproductive tract.

Good clinical practice (GCP): an ethical and scientific quality standard for designing, conducting, recording and reporting trials that involve the participation of human participants, that has its origin in the International Conference on Harmonization (ICH).[2] Compliance with this standard provides public assurance that the rights, safety and well-being of trial participants are protected, consistent with the principles that have their origin in the Declaration of Helsinki, and that the clinical trial data are credible. Although it concerns good research practices, the term clinical is used to distinguish these standards from those that apply to good laboratory and good manufacturing practices for pharmaceuticals.

---

[1] The International Development Research Centre. Module 10C: Focus Group Discussion. http://www.idrc.ca/en/ev-56615-201-1-DO_TOPIC.html (accessed 9 May 2008).

[2] International Conference on Harmonization. Guideline for Good Clinical Practice E6(R1). ICH, 1996. http://www.ich.org/cache/compo/276-254-1.html (accessed 9 May 2008)

Hepatitis B (HBV): Hepatitis is an inflammation of the liver, most commonly caused by a viral infection. There are five main hepatitis viruses, referred to as types A, B, C, D and E. Hepatitis A and E are typically caused by ingestion of contaminated food or water. Hepatitis B, C and D usually occur as a result of parenteral contact with infected body fluids (e.g. from blood transfusions or invasive medical procedures using contaminated equipment). Hepatitis B is also transmitted by sexual contact. The symptoms of hepatitis include jaundice (yellowing of the skin and eyes), dark urine, extreme fatigue, nausea, vomiting, and abdominal pain.

Histology: from the Greek "*histo*" meaning tissue, and "*logos*", meaning treatise, so histology is the scientific study of tissue.

Human rights: the "basic rights and freedoms to which all humans are entitled". Examples of rights and freedoms that are often thought of as human rights include civil and political rights, such as the right to life and liberty, freedom of expression, and equality before the law; and social, cultural, and economic rights, including the right to participate in culture, the right to food, the right to work, and the right to education. On December 10, 1948, the General Assembly of the United Nations adopted and proclaimed the Universal Declaration of Human Rights[1] as a common standard of achievement for all peoples and all nations, to the end that every individual and every organ of society, keeping this Declaration constantly in mind, shall strive by teaching and education to promote respect for these rights and freedoms and by progressive measures, national and international, to secure their universal and effective recognition and observance, both among the peoples of Member States themselves and among the peoples of territories under their jurisdiction. Some of the most important characteristics of human rights are that they are: universal; guaranteed by international standards; legally protected; focus on the dignity of the human being; and cannot be waived or taken away.

Identifiable material: includes nominal records or samples and linked, coded records or biological samples. Nominal records or samples carry a person's name or unique identifier, such as a social security number. Linked, coded records or biological samples do not carry a name but are coded and thus, by possessing or breaking the coding system, could be linked to the person to whom the record refers or from whom the sample was obtained. The code might be kept by the researcher or the sponsor or a third party.[2]

Immunity: the body's ability to protect itself against infection and disease or other unwanted biological invasion. Immunization is the process whereby a person is made immune or resistant to an infectious disease, typically by the administration of a vaccine. Vaccines stimulate the body's immune system to protect the person against subsequent infection or disease.

Immunogenic: capable of eliciting an immune response.

Innovative therapy: innovations in clinical practice which include the wide range of new diagnostic or therapeutic methods that aim to improve health outcomes beyond those of existing methods, but that have not yet been fully assessed for safety and/or efficacy. The spectrum of innovations ranges widely from minor variations of existing methods, or extension of existing methods to new indications, through to completely novel technologies.[3]

Intussusception: The bowel telescoping into itself, cutting off its own blood supply, and potentially leading to obstruction and, if untreated, death.

---

[1] Office of the High Commissioner for Human Rights. The Universal Declaration of Human Rights. http://www.ohchr.org/EN/UDHR/Pages/Introduction.aspx (accessed 9 May 2008)

[2] Council for International Organizations of Medical Sciences. International Ethical Guidelines for Epidemiological Studies. http://www.cioms.ch/frame_ethical_guidelines_2009.htm (accessed 19 May 2009)

[3] Australian National Health and Medical Research Council. Innovative Therapy or Intervention. http://www.nhmrc.gov.au/publications/hrecbook/01_commentary/13.htm (accessed 9 May 2008)

The International Conference on Harmonisation of Technical Requirements for Registration of Pharmaceuticals for Human use (ICH): a project that brings together the regulatory authorities of Europe, Japan, and the USA and experts from the pharmaceutical industry to discuss scientific and technical aspects of product registration. The Conference recommends ways to achieve greater harmonisation in the interpretation and application of technical guidelines and requirements for product registration; to facilitate a more economical use of human, animal, and material resources; to eliminate unnecessary delay in the global development and availability of new medicines; and to maintain both safeguards on quality, safety, and efficacy and regulatory obligations to protect public health.[1]

Intervention: a defined set of research activities that are implemented to achieve specified outcomes in a target population.

Intrauterine device (IUD): a small, T-shaped plastic birth-control device wrapped in copper or containing hormones, placed in the uterus. It stays effective for at least 5 years and is the most widely used contraceptive method worldwide. Intrauterine devices do not protect against sexually transmitted infections or HIV.

Investigator's brochure: a compilation of the clinical and non-clinical data on an investigational product which is relevant to the study of the product in human participants.[2]

In vitro: the technique of doing experiments in an artificial environment outside a living organism. Generally, it is performed in a laboratory.

Justice: the ethical obligation to treat each person in accordance with what is morally right and proper, and to give each person what is due to him or her. In the ethics of research involving human participants the principle refers primarily to distributive justice, which requires the equitable distribution of both the burdens and the benefits of participation in research.

Knowledge, attitude, and practice (KAP) survey: an assessment of the knowledge, attitudes, and practices of a community or group of individuals at one point in time, usually with respect to a health or health-related topic.

Malaria: a disease which can be transmitted to people of all ages. It is caused by parasites of the species *Plasmodium* that are spread from person to person through the bites of infected female *Anopheles* mosquitoes. In the human body, the parasites multiply in the liver, and then infect red blood cells. Symptoms of malaria include fever, headache, and vomiting, and usually appear between 10 and 15 days after the mosquito bite. If not treated, malaria can quickly become life-threatening by disrupting the blood supply to vital organs. In many parts of the world, the parasites have developed resistance to a number of malaria medicines. Malaria is both preventable and curable. Key interventions to control malaria include: prompt and effective treatment with artemisinin-based combination therapies; use of insecticidal nets by people at risk; and indoor residual spraying with insecticide to control the vector mosquitoes. If not treated promptly with effective medicines, malaria can cause severe illness that is often fatal. There are four types of human malaria – *P. falciparum*, *P. vivax*, *P malariae*, and *P. ovale*, The most deadly type of malaria infection is *P. falciparum*, which together with *P. vivax*, is also the most common. About 40% of the world's population, mostly those who live in the world's poorest countries, are at risk of malaria. Every year, more than 500 million people become severely ill with malaria. Most cases and deaths are in sub-Saharan Africa

---

[1] International Conference on Harmonisation of Technical Requirements for Registration of Pharmaceuticals for Human Use. http://www.ich.org/cache/compo/276-254-1.html (accessed 31 March 2008)

[2] International Conference on Harmonization. Guideline for Good Clinical Practice E6(R1). ICH, 1996. http://www.ich.org/cache/compo/276-254-1.html (accessed 9 May 2008)

Microbicide: any compound or substance whose purpose is to kill microbes (e.g. bacteria or viruses). In the context of sexually transmitted infections, microbicides are compounds that can be applied inside the vagina or rectum to protect against sexually transmitted infections including HIV. They can be formulated as gels, creams, films, or suppositories. Not all microbicides have spermicidal activity (a contraceptive effect). An effective microbicide against HIV is not yet available.

Monitoring: In the context of a clinical trial, monitoring is the act of overseeing the progress of a clinical trial, and of ensuring that it is conducted, recorded, and reported in accordance with the protocol, standard operating procedures, good clinical practice, and the applicable regulatory requirements.[1]

Multicentre trial: a clinical trial conducted according to a single protocol but at more than one site, and therefore, done by more than one investigator.[2]

Nongovernmental organization (NGO): one of a wide range of organizations that can be broadly characterized as nongovernmental, including community-based organizations (CBOs), faith-based organizations (FBOs), and organizations of affected communities.

Norfloxacin: An antibiotic used to treat many different bacterial infections.

Nuremberg Code: the first acknowledged document to lay down principles of research ethics after the war crimes tribunal at Nuremberg. It is considered to be the basic text of modern medical ethics.[3] See Permissible medical experiments on human subjects. [Nuremberg Code.] In: Trials of War Criminals Before the Nuremberg Military Tribunals under Control Council Law No 10. Vol 2, Nuremberg, October, 1946-April, 1949. Washington, DC, USA: US Government Printing.

Observational study: *see Research design*.

Oophorectomy: involves the surgical removal of a woman's ovaries in order to greatly reduce production of the estrogen and progesterone hormones which, in premenopausal women contribute to both ovarian and breast cancers.

Oral rehydration therapy (ORT): a simple, inexpensive and effective treatment for diarrhoea-related dehydration. Dehydration from diarrhoea can be prevented by giving extra fluids at home, or it can be treated simply, effectively, and cheaply in all age groups and in all but the most severe cases by giving patients an adequate oral glucose-electrolyte solution. Oral rehydration therapy, combined with guidance on appropriate feeding practices, is the main strategy recommended by WHO to reduce diarrhoea-related mortality and malnutrition in children. Oral rehydration therapy is potentially the most significant medical advance of the 20th century.

Palliative care: an approach that improves the quality of life of patients and their families who face the problems associated with life-threatening illness, through the prevention and relief of suffering by means of early identification and assessment and treatment of pain and other physical, psychosocial, and spiritual problems.

Papanicolaou (Pap) test: a routine screening test used for the detection of early cervical abnormalities, namely precancerous dysplastic changes of the uterine cervix, together with viral, bacterial, and fungal infections of the cervix and vagina. Cervical screening is a relatively simple, low-cost, and non-invasive method. Regular screening for cervical cancer reduces both the mortality from and incidence of cervical carcinoma.

---

[1] International Conference on Harmonization. Guideline for Good Clinical Practice E6(R1). Current Step 4 version. http://www.ich.org/cache/compo/276-254-1.html (accessed 9 May 2008)

[2] Ibid

[3] See Nuremberg Code. In: Trials of War Criminals Before the Nuremberg Military Tribunals under Control Council Law No 10. Vol 2, Permissible Medical Experiments on Human Subjects. Nuremberg, October, 1946-April, 1949. Washington, DC, USA: US Government Printing Office, 1949:181-182.
http://www.hhs.gov/ohrp/references/nurcode.htm (accessed 30 August 2008)

Phase I, II, III, and IV trials: The CIOMS Guidelines (see separate entry) provide useful classifications of the phases of clinical trials for vaccine development and for drug development.

In vaccine development:

- Phase I refers to the first introduction of a candidate vaccine into a human population for initial determination of its safety and biological effects, including immunogenicity. This phase can include studies of dose and route of administration, and usually involves fewer than 100 volunteers.

- Phase II refers to the initial trials to test effectiveness in about 200-500 volunteers; the focus of this phase is immunogenicity.

- Phase III trials aim to provide a more complete assessment of safety and effectiveness in the prevention of disease, and involve a larger number of volunteers, in a multicentre adequately controlled study.

In drug development:

- Phase I refers to the first introduction of a drug into humans. Normal volunteer participants are usually studied to determine the doses of drugs at which toxicity is observed. Such studies are followed by dose-ranging studies in patients for safety and, in some cases, early evidence of effectiveness.

- Phase II investigation consists of controlled clinical trials designed to demonstrate effectiveness and relative safety. Normally, these are performed on a limited number of closely monitored patients. Phase IIb proof of concept trials are now becoming more common.

- Phase III trials are performed after a reasonable probability of effectiveness of a drug has been established, and are intended to gather additional evidence of effectiveness for specific indications and more precise definition of drug-related adverse effects. This phase includes both controlled and uncontrolled studies.

- Phase IV trials are conducted after a national drug registration authority has approved a drug for distribution or marketing. These trials can include research designed to explore a specific pharmacological effect, to establish the incidence of adverse reactions, or to determine the effects of long-term administration of a drug. Phase IV trials may also be designed to evaluate a drug in a population that has not been studied adequately in the premarketing phase (such as children or the elderly) or to establish a new clinical indication for a drug. Such research is to be distinguished from marketing research, sales promotion studies, and routine post-marketing surveillance for adverse drug reactions, in that these categories ordinarily need not be reviewed by ethical review committees.[1]

Placebo: In the context of research, a placebo is a substance or procedure which patients accept as a medicine or therapy, but which actually has no specific therapeutic activity for their conditions.

---

[1] Council for International Organizations of Medical Sciences (CIOMS). International Ethical Guidelines for Biomedical Research Involving Human Subjects. Geneva, Switzerland: Council for International Organizations of Medical Sciences (CIOMS), 2002. http://www.cioms.ch (accessed 9 May 2008)

Placebo-controlled study: see **Research design**.

Plasmodium falciparum: see **Malaria**.

Plasmodium vivax: see **Malaria**.

Post traumatic stress disorder (PTSD): a psychological condition that can result from experiencing, witnessing, or participating in an overwhelmingly traumatic (frightening) event. Symptoms may include nervousness, fearfulness, poor concentration, muscle tremor and hyperventilation. Although its symptoms can occur soon after the event, the disorder often surfaces several months or even years later.

Primaquine: an 8-aminoquinoline that is effective against intrahepatic forms of all types of malaria parasite. It is used to provide radical cure of *P. vivax* and *P. ovale* malaria, in combination with a blood schizontocide for the erythrocytic parasites. Primaquine is also gametocytocidal against *P. falciparum* and has significant blood stage activity against *P. vivax* (and some against asexual stages of *P. falciparum*). The mechanism of action is unknown.[1]

Prophylactic measures: measures taken to defend against or prevent disease.

Prospective study: see **Research design**.

Public health: all organized measures (whether public or private) to prevent disease, promote health, and prolong life among the population as a whole. Its activities aim to provide conditions in which people can be healthy, and focus on entire populations, rather than individual patients or diseases. Thus, public health is concerned with the total system and not only the eradication of a particular disease.

Quinacrine hydrochloride: a dihydrochloride drug which has been used in the past as an antimalarial and for female sterilization. Various research groups (but not WHO) have attempted to exploit the sclerosing property of the antimalaria drug quinacrine for sterilization. The usual procedure is for pellets of the drug to be placed in the uterus by means of a special inserter. The pellets have been inserted in varying doses, with one, two, or three insertions, and at different times in the menstrual cycle. Insufficient data have been gathered to determine the efficacy of the method, the dosage levels needed, or the number of insertions to maximize effectiveness and minimize adverse effects. A 1992 study on efficacy showed a gross failure rate of 3.1% at 12 months after quinacrine treatment, with 40% of the patients having no menstrual period for 6 months, though 93% had resumed menstruation within one year. Although about 70 000 women have been given quinacrine for sterilization, the safety of the method remains unproven. WHO has recommended that clinical studies with quinacrine should not be undertaken until proper toxicological testing has been done.[2]

Race: a group of people connected by common descent or origin.

Randomization: The process of assigning trial participants to treatment or control groups using an element of chance to determine the assignments in order to reduce bias.[3]

Randomized control trial: see **Research design**.

Research (with human beings): any social science, biomedical, or epidemiological activity that entails systematic collection or analysis of data with the intent to generate new knowledge, in which human beings (1) are exposed to manipulation, intervention, observation, or other interaction with investigators either directly, or through alteration of their environment, or (2) become individually identifiable through investigators' collection, preparation, or use of biological material or medical or other records.

---

[1] WHO Global Malaria Programme. Guidelines for the Treatment of Malaria, 2006. http://www.who.int/malaria/treatmentguidelines.html (accessed 9 May 2008)

[2] UNDP/UNFPA/WHO/World Bank Special Programme of Research, Development and Research Training in Human Reproduction. *Progress in Reproductive Health Research* 1995. 36.
http://www.who.int/reproductive health/hrp/progress/36/news36_1.en.html (accessed 9 May 2008)

[3] International Conference on Harmonization. Guideline for Good Clinical Practice E6(R1). Geneva, Switzerland: ICH, 1996. http://www.ich.org/cache/compo/276-254-1.html (accessed 9 May 2008)

Research design: a formalized and usually systematic plan to collect data that will inform a research hypothesis.

- *Action research:* a style of research in which the researchers work with the people and for the people, rather than undertake research on them. Action research aims to generate solutions to problems identified by the people who are going to use the results of research.

- *Before-and-after study:* A control study in which results from research participants in the experimental group are compared with the outcomes from patients treated before the new intervention was available, or "historical controls".

- *Case-control study:* An observational study design that starts with the identification of individuals with the outcome of interest (such as cases of a disease) and individuals without the outcome of interest (controls). The frequencies of exposures to potential risk or protective factors for the outcome of interest are compared in cases and controls.

- *Cohort study:* a longitudinal prospective observational study in which one group of people, a "cohort", is compared over time to another group that has similar characteristics with one important difference. For example, a cohort of people who live close to a polluting factory might be compared to a cohort of people who live much further from the factory; the study might show a difference in lung capacity or asthma rates.

- *Deception research:* research in which participants are not informed about the nature of the research, or even that they are part of a research project.

- *Double-blind study:* a study design in which neither participants nor researchers know whether an individual participant is receiving the intervention being tested or a comparator (which could be either a real medical intervention or a placebo). A randomized controlled trial might be blinded, or masked, if participants in the trial could be likely to change their behaviour in a systematic way if they knew whether they had received the intervention or a comparator. The purpose of this design is to avoid unconscious subjective bias that might affect the outcome of the study. At the end of the trial, the intervention is unmasked. If problems arise in the course of the trial – specifically any danger to the health or safety of the participants – the trial will also be unmasked to ensure participants' safety.

- *Observational study:* a study design in which investigators observe and record events.

- *Placebo-controlled study:* a research design in which a "dummy" or inert intervention is used as a comparator in a control arm of the study in order to eliminate bias.

- *Prospective study:* a study in which data on exposures and disease outcome are collected as the events occur, unlike a retrospective study.

- *Randomized controlled study (RCT):* a design in which participants are randomly assigned either to an intervention group (e.g. a drug treatment) or to a control group (e.g. a placebo or an active comparator). Both groups are monitored over a specific period of time and the effects of the intervention on specific outcomes (dependent variables) defined at the outset are analysed (e.g. serum cholesterol levels, death rates, or remission rates).

- *Retrospective study:* a study in which data on exposures and disease outcome are collected some time after the event, unlike a prospective study. Also refers to an observational study design in which the investigators study both present and past events

- *Single-blind study:* a study design in which the investigator, but not the participant, knows the treatment assignment.

Resection: the full or partial surgical removal of any tissue or organ.

Respect for persons: incorporates at least two fundamental ethical considerations, namely:

a respect for autonomy, which requires that those who are capable of deliberation about their personal choices should be treated with respect for their capacity for self-determination; and

b protection of people with impaired or diminished autonomy, which requires that those who are dependent or vulnerable be afforded security against harm or abuse.[1]

Risk factor: any attribute, characteristic, or exposure of an individual, which increases the likelihood of developing a disease or injury.

Retrospective study: *see Research design.*

Severe acute respiratory syndrome (SARS): a viral respiratory illness that can cause death, caused by a coronavirus (SARS CoV). Initial symptoms are similar to influenza, including a fever, and usually appear 2-10 days after exposure (but can appear up to 13 days later). In most cases, symptoms appear within 2-3 days. SARS CoV is believed to be an animal virus that crossed the species barrier to humans recently when ecological changes or changes in human behaviour increased opportunities for human exposure to the virus and virus adaptation, enabling human-to-human transmission.

By July, 2003, the international spread of SARS CoV resulted in 8098 SARS cases in 26 countries, with 774 deaths. The epidemic created pressures on health services and caused social and economic disruption, especially in areas with sustained local transmission of SARS; it also affected the international travel industry.[2]

Schizophrenia: a mental disorder, characterized by profound disruptions in thinking, affecting language, perception, and the sense of self. It often includes psychotic experiences, such as hearing voices or delusions. It can impair functioning through the loss of an acquired capability to earn a livelihood or the disruption of studies. Schizophrenia typically begins in late adolescence or early adulthood. Most cases of schizophrenia can be treated, and people affected by it can lead a productive life and be integrated in society.

Sclerosing agent: A substance that causes marked tissue irritation and/or clotting inside a blood vessel, with subsequent local inflammation and tissue destruction.

Serious adverse event (SAE) or Serious adverse drug reaction (serious ADR): Any untoward medical occurrence that at any dose results in death, is life-threatening, requires inpatient hospitalization or prolongation of existing hospitalization, results in persistent or significant disability/incapacity, or is a congenital anomaly or birth defect.[3]

---

[1] Council for International Organizations of Medical Sciences (CIOMS). International Ethical Guidelines for Biomedical Research Involving Human Subjects. Geneva, Switzerland: Council for International Organizations of Medical Sciences (CIOMS), 2002. http://www.cioms.ch (accessed 9 May 2008)

[2] WHO. WHO Guidelines for the Global Surveillance of Severe Acute Respiratory Syndrome (SARS). Updated Recommendations, October 2004. http://www.who.int/csr/resources/publications/WHO_CDS_CSR_ARO_2004_1/en/index.html (accessed 9 May 2008)

[3] International Conference on Harmonization. Guideline for Good Clinical Practice E6(R1). Geneva, Switzerland: ICH, 1996. http://www.ich.org/cache/compo/276-254-1.html (accessed 9 May 2008)

Sexually transmitted infection (STI): an infection that is spread primarily through person-to-person sexual contact. There are more than 30 different sexually transmissible bacteria, viruses and parasites. The most common conditions they cause are gonorrhoea, chlamydial infection, syphilis, trichomoniasis, chancroid, genital herpes, genital warts, human immunodeficiency virus (HIV) infection, and hepatitis B infection. Several, in particular HIV and syphilis, can also be transmitted from mother to child during pregnancy and childbirth, and through blood products and tissue transfer.

Single-blind study: *see Research design.*

Somatoform disorders: a group of mental disturbances placed in a common category on the basis of their external symptoms. These disorders are characterized by physical complaints that appear to be medical in origin but that cannot be explained in terms of a physical disease, the results of substance abuse, or by another mental disorder.

Sponsor: an individual, company, institution, or organization which takes responsibility for the initiation, management, and/or financing of research.[1]

Squamous intraepithelial lesion (SIL): a general term for the abnormal growth of squamous cells on the surface of the cervix. The changes in the cells are described as low grade (LSIL) or high grade (HSIL), depending on how much of the cervix is affected and how abnormal the cells are.[2] HSIL is regarded as a significant precancerous lesion, whereas low-grade SIL (LSIL) is more benign, since most of these lesions regress.[3]

Standard operating procedures (SOPs): detailed, written instructions to achieve uniformity of the performance of a specific function.[4] A research ethics committee, for example, should have standard operating procedures to guide its role.

Stem cells: unspecialized cells that renew themselves for long periods through cell division and have the remarkable potential to develop into many different cell types in the body. Typically they serve as the repair system for the body and are found in the bone marrow in adults and can be obtained from the umbilical cord. Under certain physiological or experimental conditions, they can be induced to become cells with special functions such as the beating cells of the heart muscle or the insulin-producing cells of the pancreas.[5]

Stigma: a process of producing and reproducing inequitable power relations, whereby inequalities in society are created and sustained through negative attitudes towards a group of people on the basis of particular attributes such as their HIV status, gender, sexuality, or behaviour.

Structured interview: an interview, generally with only one interviewee, in which questions are predefined and asked in a specific order, and the interviewer or an assistant records the answers.

Surveillance: In the context of public health, the ongoing systematic collection, collation, analysis, and interpretation of data, with dissemination of information to those who need to know in order that action may be taken.

Tamoxifen: an anti-oestrogenic drug, tamoxifen has been used for almost two decades as the first-line endocrine therapy for postmenopausal women who have advanced metastatic breast cancer. Tamoxifen is also used as adjuvant therapy in patients with breast cancer and is being tested for use as a preventive agent. There is conclusive evidence that tamoxifen reduces the risk for contralateral breast cancer in women with a previous diagnosis of breast cancer.

Teratogen: Any medication, chemical, infectious disease, or environmental agent that might interfere with the normal development of a fetus and result in the loss of a pregnancy, a birth defect, or a pregnancy complication.

---

[1] International Conference on Harmonization. Guideline for Good Clinical Practice E6(R1). Op. cit.

[2] National Cancer Institute. http://www.cancer.gov/Templates/db_alpha.aspx?CdrID=46596 (accessed 9 May 2008)

[3] Saslow D, Runowicz CD, Solomon D, et al; American Cancer Society. American Cancer Society Guideline for the Early Detection of Cervical Neoplasia and Cancer. *CA Cancer J Clin* 2002; 52: 342-62.

[4] International Conference on Harmonization. Guideline for Good Clinical Practice E6(R1). Op. cit.

[5] US National Institutes of Health. Stem Cell Basics. http://stemcells.nih.gov/info/basics/basics1.asp (accessed 9 May 2008)

Tetanus: a disease caused by the bacterium *Clostridium tetani*. It is characterized by muscle spasms, initially in the jaw muscles. As the disease progresses, mild stimuli can trigger generalized tetanic seizure-like activity, which contributes to serious complications and eventually death unless supportive treatment is given. Tetanus can be prevented by the administration of tetanus toxoid, which induces specific antitoxins. To prevent maternal and neonatal tetanus, tetanus toxoid needs to be given to the mother before or during pregnancy, and clean delivery and cord care needs to be ensured.

Triage: the process of selecting for care or for treatment those of highest priority or, when resources are limited, those who are more likely to benefit.[1]

Trichomonas vaginalis: a sexually transmitted infection, and the most common pathogenic protozoan infection of women in industrialized countries.

TRIPS: The Agreement on Trade-Related Aspects of Intellectual Property Rights (TRIPS), a basic document adopted in 1994 by the World Trade Organization (WTO), establishes obligations of Member Nations to enforce patents and other intellectual property rights. The TRIPS Agreement permits "compulsory licensing", which is "authorization, given by a government, to use a patented invention without the consent of the patent-holder" upon payment of a small royalty, in order to allow a country to provide treatments that would otherwise be unavailable because of the patent. For more information, visit http://www.wto.org/english/tratop_e/trips_e/t_agm1_e.htm

Tubal occlusion: a surgical procedure for permanently terminating a woman's fertility by blocking the fallopian tubes (via tying and cutting, rings, clips or electrocautery), preventing sperm from reaching the ova and causing fertilization.

Tuberculosis (TB): an infectious bacterial disease caused by *Mycobacterium tuberculosis*, which most commonly affects the lungs. It is transmitted from person to person via droplets from the throat and lungs of people with the active respiratory disease. In healthy people, infection with *M tuberculosis* often causes no symptoms, since the person's immune system acts to "wall off" the bacteria. The symptoms of active tuberculosis of the lung are coughing, sometimes with sputum or blood, chest pain, weakness, weight loss, fever, and night sweats. Tuberculosis is treatable with a 6-month course of antibiotics

Vasectomy: Surgical method of male sterilization by removal of sections from each *vas deferens*.

Vertical transmission: Spread of infection from the mother directly to the offspring during pregnancy, birth, or breastfeeding.

Vulnerable (research) participants: Individuals whose willingness to volunteer in a clinical trial (or other type of research) might be unduly influenced by the expectation, whether justified or not, of benefits associated with participation, or of a retaliatory response from senior members of a hierarchy in case of refusal to participate. Examples are members of a group with a hierarchical structure, such as medical, pharmacy, dental, and nursing students, subordinate hospital and laboratory personnel, employees of the pharmaceutical industry, members of the armed forces, and people kept in detention. Other vulnerable participants could include patients with incurable diseases, people in nursing homes, unemployed or impoverished people, patients in emergency situations, ethnic minority groups, homeless people, nomads, refugees, minors, and those incapable of giving consent.[2] This list might not be exhaustive, since in some circumstances other groups are considered vulnerable (e.g. women in an orthodox patriarchical society).

Whistleblowing: reporting misconduct of an organization, such as violations of the law, corruption, fraud, or health and safety violations. The term is usually used to describe the action taken by an employee when making such misconduct public, especially within a business or government agency.

---

[1] Last J. A Dictionary of Epidemiology. 4th edition. Oxford, UK: Oxford University Press, 2001.

[2] International Conference on Harmonization. Guideline for Good Clinical Practice E6(R1). Geneva, Switzerland: ICH, 1996.

Suggested readings and resources

The readings and resources listed here are organized under the following headings:

1. Those related to guidelines and guidance on ethics regulations
2. Literature on Ethics Review Committees
3. Literature on ethics and international health research
4. Suggested reading by chapter (this reading list also appears at the end of each chapter)

   - Chapter I Defining "Research": When must an ethics committee's approval be sought?
   - Chapter II Issues in Study Design: Designing scientifically (and ethically) sound studies
   - Chapter III Harm, Benefit and Just Allocation: Are research benefits and harms fairly distributed?
   - Chapter IV Informed Consent: Is consent to research voluntary, knowing, and competent?
   - Chapter V Standard of Care: Whose standard?
   - Chapter VI Obligations to Participants and Communities: How far do researchers' and sponsors' duties extend?
   - Chapter VII Privacy and Confidentiality: Why control access to information?
   - Chapter VIII Professional Ethics: Conflicts of interest and scientific misconduct

Selected guidelines and guidance documents

In this section, several key international guidance documents are identified and briefly described. Many regional, national, local, and institutional guidance documents have also been developed, but they are far too numerous to include here. However, researchers and ethics committee members should not only be aware of and adhere to international guidance, but also the guidance which is applicable in their own regional, national, and local research contexts. For example, if a researcher is conducting HIV/AIDS vaccine research with an indigenous population in country X, they should honour both international and country-specific guidelines, and any special provisions or guidance developed for research with that community.

In addition to these specific guidance documents, there are laws, regulations, and required procedures which might not be presented in the form of sets of guidelines or coherent documents for research guidance, but which are, nevertheless, crucial in the conduct of research which is ethical and legal. These laws, regulations, and procedures might not always be easy to locate but, increasingly, there are resources to assist with this. Four websites might be of interest:

- The Global Research Ethics Map (GREmap) is an online resource which presents legal, regulatory, and procedural guidance on a country-by-country basis. GREmap is developed and maintained by the Harvard School of Public Health. https://webapps.sph.harvard.edu/live/gremap/index_main.cfm (accessed 30 March 2008)

- The United States Department of Health and Human Services, Office for Human Research Protection (OHRP) has developed an "International Compilation of Human Research Protections" which provides a listing of the laws, regulations, and guidelines that govern research with human participants in 84 countries around the world.
  http://hhs.gov/ohrp/international/HSPCompilation.pdf (accessed 9 May 2008)

- TRREE for Africa (Training and Resources in Research Ethics Evaluation for Africa) is a web-based training and capacity-building initiative on the ethics of research with humans conducted in Africa countries. Distance learning on evaluation of research ethics is being made freely available through this bilingual (French-English) initiative, which is also developing a participatory website of international, regional, and national regulatory and policy resources.
  http://www.trree.org/site/en_home.phtml (accessed 30 March 2008).

- United Nations Educational, Scientific and Cultural Organization (UNESCO) is actively engaged in bioethics in a range of capacities including the development of universal declarations on bioethics and human rights (see separate Guidelines section). UNESCO's Global Ethics Observatory provides a number of ethics-related databases, one of which is devoted to regulations and guidelines related to research ethics in various countries.
http://portal.unesco.org/shs/en/ev.php-URL_ID=11277&URL_DO=DO_TOPIC&URL_SECTION=201.html (accessed 9 May 2008)

CIOMS. International Ethical Guidelines for Biomedical Research Involving Human Subjects. Geneva, Switzerland: Council for International Organizations of Medical Sciences (CIOMS), 2002.

The CIOMS (Council for International Organizations of Medical Science) Guidelines, properly titled International Ethical Guidelines for Biomedical Research Involving Human Subjects, are "designed to be of use to countries in defining national policies on the ethics of biomedical research involving human subjects, applying ethical standards in local circumstances, and establishing or improving ethical review mechanisms. A particular aim is to reflect the conditions and the needs of low-resource countries, and the implications for multinational or transnational research in which they may be partners." Like the Declaration of Helsinki, the CIOMS Guidelines provide important guidance on the ethical conduct of health research. The guidelines were prepared by CIOMS in collaboration with WHO.

http://www.cioms.ch (accessed 9 May 2008)

CIOMS. International Ethical Guidelines for Epidemiological Studies. Geneva, Switzerland: Council for International Organizations of Medical Sciences (CIOMS), 2009.

The CIOMS (Council for International Organizations of Medical Science) Guidelines for Epidemiological Studies "provides ethical guidance for epidemiologists, as well as those who sponsor, review, or participate in epidemiological studies, on identifying and responding to the ethical issues that are raised by the process of producing this knowledge." The guidelines were prepared by CIOMS in collaboration with WHO.

http://www.cioms.ch (accessed 19 May 2009)

Council of Europe. Convention for the Protection of Human Rights and Dignity of the Human Being with regard to the Application of Biology and Medicine: Convention on Human Rights and Biomedicine. Strasbourg, France: Council of Europe, 1997.

Also known as the Oviedo convention, this European document is a binding legal instrument designed to safeguard human dignity and fundamental rights against any improper applications of medicine and biology. It has been adopted by the Council of Europe's Committee of Ministers and has been signed by 21 European countries.

http://conventions.coe.int/treaty/en/treaties/html/164.htm (accessed 9 May 2008)

International Conference on Harmonisation of Technical Requirements for Registration of Pharmaceuticals for Human Use (ICH). ICH Harmonised Tripartite Guideline. Guideline for Good Practice. Geneva, Switzerland: ICH Secretariat, International Federation for Pharmaceutical Manufacturers Association, 1996.

"The objective of this ICH GCP Guideline, is to provide a unified standard for the European Union (EU), Japan and the United States, to facilitate the mutual acceptance of clinical data by the regulatory authorities in these jurisdictions. [...] The guideline should be followed when generating clinical trial data that are intended to be submitted to regulatory authorities. The principles established in this guideline may also be applied to other clinical investigation that may have an impact on the safety and well-being of human subjects."

http://www.ich.org/LOB/media/MEDIA482.pdf (accessed 9 May 2008)

National Bioethics Advisory Commission. Ethical and Policy Issues in International Research: Clinical Trials in Developing Countries, Volumes I and II. Bethesda, MD, USA: National Bioethics Advisory Commission, 2001.

These two volumes report on the findings – background and recommendations – from the NBAC, an American commission which examined numerous ethical issues which arise when research is conducted in developing or resource-poor countries but sponsored and conducted by U.S. interests abroad.

http://bioethics.georgetown.edu/nbac/pubs.html (accessed 9 May 2008)

National Commission for the Protection of Human Subjects of Biomedical and Behavioural Research. The Belmont Report: Ethical Principles and Guidelines for the Protection of Human Subjects of Research. Washington, DC, USA: Department of Health, Education, and Welfare, 1979.

Based on the deliberations of the commission, this report serves as an important historical document in the development of research ethics and it remains relevant for its clarity in presenting certain basic ethical principles and definitions (respect for persons, justice and beneficence, for example) and their procedural application.

http://bioethics.georgetown.edu/nrc/archives/ncphsguide.pdf (accessed 9 May 2008)

Nuffield Council on Bioethics. The Ethics of Research Related to Healthcare in Developing Countries. London, UK: Nuffield Foundation, 2002.

This report "examines the ethical issues raised when research related to healthcare is carried out in developing countries and funded by sponsors from developed countries" and offers ways forward. Consent, standards of care, post research obligations and ethical oversight are discussed knowledgeably and in-depth. The report emphasizes the importance of enhancing the ability of developing countries to conduct research that is relevant to their needs.

http://www.nuffieldbioethics.org/go/ourwork/developingcountries/introduction (accessed 9 May 2008)

Nuffield Council on Bioethics. The Ethics of Research Related to Healthcare in Developing Countries: A Follow-up Discussion Paper. London, UK: Nuffield Foundation, 2005.

This discussion paper provides additional points for consideration that arose subsequent to the publication of the Nuffield Council Report of the same name. The paper explores the practical implications resulting from the revision of several international guidelines and the development of others.

http://www.nuffieldbioethics.org/go/ourwork/developingcountries/page_246.html (accessed 9 May 2008)

UNAIDS/WHO. Ethical Considerations in Biomedical HIV Prevention Trials – UNAIDS/WHO guidance document. Geneva, Switzerland: Joint United Nations Programme on HIV/AIDS (UNAIDS) and the World Health Organization, 2007.

This publication updates the UNAIDS guidance document titled 'Ethical considerations in HIV preventive vaccine research' (2000). The revision outlines 19 guidance points and incorporates developments which have taken place since the original publication, including new aspects regarding biomedical HIV-prevention research.

http://whqlibdoc.who.int/unaids/2007/9789291736256_eng.pdf (accessed 25 August 2008)

UNAIDS/AVAC. Good Participatory Practice Guidelines for Biomedical HIV Prevention Trials. Geneva, Switzerland: Joint United Nations Programme on HIV/AIDS (UNAIDS) and the AIDS Vaccine Advisory Council (AVAC), 2007.

This publication complements the 'Ethical Considerations in biomedical HIV prevention trials – UNAIDS/WHO guidance document' and aims to provide systematic guidance on the engagement with communities that research entities should strive for by examining the roles and responsibilities of those entities, as well as the roles and responsibilities of the communities themselves in the research process.

http://whqlibdoc.who.int/unaids/2007/9789291736348_eng.pdf (accessed 25 August 2008)

UNESCO. International Declaration on Human Genetic Data. Paris: United Nations Educational, Scientific and Cultural Organization, 2003.

"In the [rapidly developing field of genetic research], many people fear that human genetic data will be used for purposes contrary to human rights and freedom." Together with the Universal Declaration on the Human Genome and Human Rights, and the Universal Declaration on Bioethics and Human Rights, these guidelines provide important international points of reference in the field of bioethics, bearing in mind the protection of human rights and fundamental freedoms and stressing that all medical data should be treated with the same high standards of confidentiality.

http://portal.unesco.org/shs/en/ev.php-URL_ID=1882&URL_DO=DO_TOPIC&URL_SECTION=201.html (accessed 9 May 2008)

UNESCO. Universal Declaration on Bioethics and Human Rights. Paris, France: United Nations Educational, Scientific and Cultural Organization, 2005.

This Universal Declaration commits UNESCO member states and the international community to "respect and apply the fundamental principles of bioethics set forth within a single text. [...] By enshrining bioethics in international human rights, and by ensuring respect for the life of human beings, the Declaration recognizes the interrelation between ethics and human rights in the specific field of bioethics."

http://portal.unesco.org/shs/en/ev.php-URL_ID=1883&URL_DO=DO_TOPIC&URL_SECTION=201.html (accessed 9 May 2008)

UNESCO. Universal Declaration on the Human Genome and Human Rights. Paris, France: United Nations Educational, Scientific and Cultural Organization, 1997.

This declaration is the first universal instrument in the field of bioethics. Its aim is to establish a balance between safeguarding respect for human rights and fundamental freedoms and ensuring freedom of research. It serves as a document committing states to take appropriate measures to promote these principles, constituting the beginning of international awareness of the need of ethics in science and technology.

http://portal.unesco.org/shs/en/ev.php-URL_ID=2228&URL_DO=DO_TOPIC&URL_SECTION=201.html (accessed 9 May 2008)

WHO. *Guidelines for Good Clinical Practice (GCP) for Trials on Pharmaceutical Products* **(Annex 3) in The Use of Essential Drugs: Sixth Report of the WHO Expert Committee. Geneva, Switzerland: World Health Organization, 1995**

The purpose of these guidelines is to set globally applicable standards for the conduct of biomedical research trials on pharmaceutical products with human subjects. "By providing a basis both for the scientific and ethical integrity of research involving human subjects and for generating valid observations and sound documentation of the findings, these Guidelines not only serve the interests of the parties actively involved in the research process, but protect the rights and safety of subjects, including patients, and ensure that the investigations are directed to the advancement of public health objectives."

http://whqlibdoc.who.int/trs/WHO_TRS_850.pdf (accessed 25 August 2008)

WHO. Handbook for Good Clinical Research Practice (GCP), Guidance for Implementation. Geneva, Switzerland: World Health Organization, 2005.

"This handbook is an adjunct to WHO's Guidelines for good clinical practice (GCP) for trials on pharmaceutical products (1995), and is intended to assist national regulatory authorities, sponsors, investigators and ethics committees in implementing GCP for industry-sponsored, government-sponsored, institution-sponsored, or investigator-initiated clinical research. The handbook is based on international guidelines and is organized as a reference and educational tool to facilitate understanding and implementation of GCP."

http://whqlibdoc.who.int/publications/2005/924159392X_eng.pdf (accessed 25 August 2008)

WHO. Operational Guidelines for Ethics Committees that Review Biomedical Research. Geneva, Switzerland: World Health Organization, 2000.

This book sets out operational guidelines for ethics committees in order to facilitate, support, and ensure quality of the ethical review of biomedical research in all countries around the world. Targeted for use by national and local bodies, these guidelines define the role and constituents of an ethics committee, and detail the requirements for submitting an application for review. The review procedure and details of the decision making process are provided, as well as necessary follow-up and documentation procedures.

http://whqlibdoc.who.int/hq/2000/TDR_PRD_ETHICS_2000.1.pdf (accessed 25 August 2008)

WHO. Putting Women First: Ethical and Safety Recommendations for Research on Domestic Violence Against Women. Geneva, Switzerland: World Health Organization, 2001.

This publication offers recommendations on the ethical conduct of domestic violence research. The recommendations are designed for anyone intending to do research on domestic violence against women, and also for those initiating or reviewing such research.

http://whqlibdoc.who.int/hq/2001/WHO_FCH_GWH_01.1.pdf (accessed 25 August 2008)

WHO. WHO Ethical and Safety Recommendations for Researching, Documenting and Monitoring Sexual Violence in Emergencies. Geneva, Switzerland: World Health Organization, 2007.

"Sexual violence in humanitarian emergencies, such as armed conflict and natural disasters, is a serious, even life-threatening, public health and human rights issue". The eight recommendations offered in this publication are intended to ensure that before commencing any information gathering exercise concerning sexual violence in emergencies, the necessary safety and ethical safeguards are in place.

http://whqlibdoc.who.int/publications/2007/9789241595681_eng.pdf (accessed 25 August 2008)

World Medical Association. Declaration of Helsinki: Ethical Principles for Medical Research Involving Human Subjects. Helsinki, Finland: World Medical Association, 1964. Latest revised and updated version 2008.

This declaration by the World Medical Association (WMA) serves as a statement of ethical principles to provide guidance to physicians and others involved in medical research with human beings and identifiable human material or identifiable data. It is one of the most widely known and accepted guideline documents for research ethics. Amendments and clarifications have been made to the original 1964 Declaration and the WMA stresses that the most recent version is the only one in effect.

http://www.wma.net/e/ethicsunit/helsinki.htm (accessed 5 June 2009)

World Trade Organization. The Agreement on Trade-Related Aspects of Intellectual Property Rights. Geneva, Switzerland: World Trade Organization, 1994.

"TRIPS" is a document adopted in 1994 by the World Trade Organization (WTO), which establishes obligations of Member Nations to enforce patents and other intellectual property rights. The TRIPS Agreement permits "compulsory licensing", which is "authorization, given by a government, to use a patented invention without the consent of the patent-holder" upon payment of a small royalty, in order to allow a country to provide treatments that would otherwise be unavailable because of the patent.

http://www.wto.org/english/tratop_e/trips_e/t_agm1_e.htm (accessed 30 August 2008)

Research ethics committees

Bhutta ZA. Building Capacity for Ethical Review in Developing Countries. *Science and Development Network*, 2004

"The need for case-by-case review of proposed medical research has been on the international agenda for several decades. But the main operational mechanism used to ensure that clinical research conforms to ethical standards, and that participants in such research are protected – in the form of research ethics committees (RECs) – is still inadequate in the developing world." Zulfiqar A Bhutta sets out the constraints faced by members of RECs in developing countries, and offers suggestions to improve the situation.

http://www.scidev.net/en/policy-briefs/building-capacity-for-ethical-review-in-developing.html (accessed 9 May 2008)

Emanuel EJ, Lemmens T, Elliot C. Should Society Allow Research Ethics Boards to be Run as For-profit Enterprises? *PLoS Medicine*, 2006, 3(7).

"Traditionally, IRBs [or ethics committees] have been run by volunteer committees of scientists and clinicians working in the academic medical centers where the studies they review are being carried out. However, for-profit organizations are increasingly being hired to conduct ethics reviews." Presented as a debate between the pros and cons of for-profit ethics committees, the authors succinctly address the issues and evidence in their opposing arguments.

http://dx.doi.org/10.1371/journal.pmed.0030309 (accessed 25 August 2008)

Eckstein S. Efforts to Build Capacity in Research Ethics: An Overview. *Science and Development Network*, 2004.

"During the past five years there has been a dramatic increase in the number and type of initiatives to build capacity in research ethics in developing countries. In this policy brief Sue Eckstein gives an overview of such initiatives, and indicates that there is unlikely to be a "best way" to build capacity. Instead, many different routes may lead to enhanced levels of understanding about research ethics." This article is online only.

http://www.scidev.net/en/science-and-innovation-policy/research-ethics/policy-briefs/efforts-to-build-capacity-in-research-ethics-an-ov.html (accessed 9 May 2008)

Kass NE, et al. The Structure and Function of Research Ethics Committees in Africa: A Case Study. *PLoS Medicine*, 2007;4:1.

"This case study examines the history, operations, strengths, and challenges of 12 African RECs. [The authors] hope this will help researchers working in Africa better understand the landscape of ethics review and help funders target resources for capacity development in a continent where health research is so critical to development, and local responsibility for research functions is critical for research."

http://dx.doi.org/10.1371/journal.pmed.0040003 (accessed 25 August 2008)

Loff B, Black J. Research Ethics Committees: What Is Their Contribution? *Medical Journal of Australia*, 2004;181(8).

"Perhaps a week of intensive training in critical thinking would be the best preparation for members of research ethics committees. Perhaps we all must consider how best to deal with situations about which not all agree, and about which objections are morally relevant. Furthermore, there are many issues that are not well addressed by guidelines or law."

http://www.mja.com.au/public/issues/181_08_181004/lof10613_fm.html (accessed 9 May 2008)

Ethics and international health-related research

Beauchamp T, Childress J. Principles of Biomedical Ethics, 5th Edition. New York, USA: Oxford University Press, 2001.

A foundational text on moral and ethical reasoning in biomedical ethics. Four core chapters on the ethical principles of respect for autonomy, non-maleficence, justice, and beneficence provide the framework for their reasoning. This latest edition has been updated to reflect current issues, examples, and arguments.

Benatar S. Reflections and Recommendations in Research Ethics in Developing Countries. *Social Science & Medicine*, 2002;54:1131-1141.

This publication discusses the global context in which debates on the ethics of international clinical research, particularly the issues regarding informed consent and the distribution of benefits and of harm to individual and communities, take place. The author proposes a wider role for research ethics committees and new ways of thinking about the role of research ethics

http://www.equinetafrica.org/bibl/docs/BENmon.pdf
(accessed 9 May 2008)

Beyrer C, Kass NE. Human Rights, Politics, and Reviews of Research Ethics. *Lancet*, 2002, 360:246-251.

"Every element of a research ethics review – the balance of risks and benefits, the assurance of rights for individual participants, and the fair selection of research populations – can be affected by the political and human rights background in which a study is done. Research that at first seems to be low in risk may become high in risk if implemented in a country where the government might breach the confidentiality of study results or where results might be used to deport a refugee group." This paper draws attention to the importance of understanding the political and human rights background of the setting in which studies are being carried out. The authors argue that researchers must take these problems into account before deciding to do research in a given setting.

http://dx.doi.org/10.1016/S0140-6736(02)09465-5
(accessed 25 August 2008)

Emanuel EJ, et al. What Makes Clinical Research in Developing Countries Ethical? The Benchmarks of Ethical Research. *Journal of Infectious Diseases*, 2004, 189:932-937.

"Research in developing countries creates a greater risk of exploitation: individuals or communities in developing countries assume the risks of research, but most of the benefits may accrue to people in developed countries". The authors of this publication apply a previously proposed ethical framework for clinical research within developing countries and propose practical guidelines for researchers and research-ethics committees.

http://dx.doi.org/10.1086/381709
(accessed 25 August 2008)

Lavery JV, et al. Ethical Issues in International Biomedical Research: A Casebook. Oxford, UK: Oxford University Press, 2007.

This compilation of 21 international biomedical research case studies is accompanied by commentaries from bioethicists, researchers, and other experts, including many in developing countries, which encourage readers to appreciate divergent approaches and perspectives to a wide range of ethical issues. The case studies are organized by issue (for example, 'favourable risk-benefit ratio', 'informed consent', and 'respect for enrolled subjects and study communities') and are very useful additions to the suggested chapter-by-chapter readings listed below.

Tan-Torres Edejer, T. North-South Research Partnerships: the Ethics of Carrying out Research in Developing Countries. *British Medical Journal*, 1999;319:438-441.

This article focuses on the problems, and the possibilities, arising in North-South research collaborations. The author argues that health research is a public good, and that, as such, the burden and benefits of research should be shared by both the North and South partners. In addition, the measure of success should not be the narrow focus of scientific advances but must include "the choice of identified priorities as areas of work, the sustainability of the studied interventions outside the research setting, and the investment in local research capacity…".

http://www.bmj.com/cgi/content/extract/319/7207/438
(accessed 10 May 2008)

Suggested readings by chapter

I. Defining "Research"

Centers for Disease Control and Prevention. Guidelines for Defining Public Health Research and Public Health Non-Research. Revised October 4, 1999. Atlanta, GA, USA: CDC, 1999.

This document "sets forth CDC guidelines on the definition of public health research conducted by CDC staff irrespective of the funding source (i.e. provided by CDC or by another entity). Under Federal regulations (45 CFR 46), the final determination of what is research and whether the Federal regulations are applicable lies with CDC and, ultimately, with the Office for Protection from Research Risks (OPRR)." The guidance is intended for use by state and local health departments and other institutions that conduct collaborative research with CDC staff or that are recipients of CDC funds.

http://www.cdc.gov/od/science/regs/hrpp/researchDefinition.htm (accessed 9 May 2008)

Wade DT. Ethics, Audit, and Research: All Shades of Grey. *British Medical Journal*, 2005, 330: 468-471.

"All research studies have to be scrutinized by an ethics committee […] but most ethics committees specifically exclude audit studies from their remit. Similarly, journal editors and funding agencies will require evidence of ethical review before accepting research for publication or funding but do not require this for audit studies. Consequently, the distinction between audit and research can have important implications, and the temptation to label research as audit is considerable." This article reviews the difficult distinction between audit and research, and includes four illustrative case studies which readers are invited to analyze and respond to.

http://dx.doi.org/10.1136/bmj.330.7489.468
(accessed 25 August 2008)

II. Issues in Study Design

Allmark P, Mason S. Should Desperate Volunteers be Included in Randomized Controlled Trials? *Journal of Medical Ethics* 2006;32:548-553.

"Randomised controlled trials (RCTs) sometimes recruit participants who are desperate to receive the experimental treatment. This paper defends the practice against three arguments that suggest it is unethical first, desperate volunteers are not in equipoise. Second clinicians, entering patients onto trials are disavowing their therapeutic obligation to deliver the best treatment; they are following trial protocols rather than delivering individualised care. […] Third, desperate volunteers do not give proper consent: effectively, they are coerced."

http://dx.doi.org/10.1136/jme.2005.014282
(accessed 25 August 2008)

Marshall PA. Ethical Challenges in Study Design and Informed Consent for Health Research in Resource-poor Settings. Geneva, Switzerland: WHO/TDR, 2007.

"This review considers ethical challenges to research design and informed consent in biomedical and behavioural studies conducted in resource-poor settings. A review of the literature explores relevant social, cultural, and ethical issues in the conduct of biomedical and social health research in developing countries. Ten case vignettes illustrate ethical challenges that arise in international research with culturally diverse populations." Recommendations are offered to researchers and policy-makers concerned with ethical practices in multinational studies conducted in resource-poor settings.

https://www.who.int/tdr/publications/tdr-research-publications/ethical-challenges-study-design/pdf/ethical_challenges.pdf
(accessed 30 August 2008)

Van den Borne F. Using Mystery Clients to Assess Condom Negotiation in Malawi: Some Ethical Concerns. *Studies in Family Planning* 2007;38[4].

"Although most international ethical research codes prescribe the informed consent of research Subjects, the present author, as principal investigator for that study, included the mystery client method, which omits informants' consent. […] This article is intended to contribute to the dialogue and debate on ethical research involving mystery clients and to encourage other researchers to share their ethical dilemmas and show how they have addressed them."

http://dx.doi.org/10.1111/j.1728-4465.2007.00144.x
(accessed 25 August 2008)

Weiger C, et al. For and against: Clinical Equipoise and Not the Uncertainty Principle is the Moral Underpinning of the Randomised Controlled Trial. *British Medical Journal*, 2000; 321:756-758.

"The ethical basis for entering patients in randomised controlled trials is under debate. Some doctors espouse the uncertainty principle whereby randomisation to treatment is acceptable when an individual doctor is genuinely unsure which treatment is best for a patient. Others believe that clinical equipoise, reflecting collective professional uncertainty over treatment, is the soundest ethical criterion." While uncertainty is a basic ethical requirement principle for RCTs, this article debates what is meant by uncertainty in a research context.

http://dx.doi.org/10.1136/bmj.321.7263.756
(accessed 25 August 2008)

III. Harm and Benefit

Bayer A, Tadd W. Unjustified Exclusion of Elderly People from Studies Submitted to Ethics Committees for Approval: Descriptive Study. *British Medical Journal*, 2000; 321:992-993.

"Ethics committees are in a strong position to influence research practice and to reduce unethical age discrimination. We encourage them to request justification whenever protocols include inappropriate age restrictions – and if this is not forthcoming, approval might be conditional on age limits being removed. This policy would promote more positive attitudes towards elderly people among researchers as well as safer, more effective treatments and services."

http://dx.doi.org/10.1136/bmj.321.7267.992
(accessed 25 August 2008)

Moodley K. Microbicide Research in Developing Countries: Have We Given the Ethical Concerns Due Consideration? *BioMedCentral Medical Ethics*, 2007; 8:10

"Ethical concerns relating to safety in microbicide research are a major international concern. However, in the urgency to develop a medically efficacious microbicide, some of these concerns may not have been anticipated. In the risk-benefit assessment of research protocols, both medical and psycho-social risk must be considered." This article examines a number of concerns related to safety risks in international microbicide trials.

http://dx.doi.org/10.1186/1472-6939-8-10
(accessed 25 August 2008)

Schenk K, Williamson J. Ethical Approaches to Gathering Information from Children and Adolescents in International Settings – Guidelines and Approaches. Washington, DC, USA: Population Council, 2005.

"Program managers and researchers often gather information from children and adolescents in order to develop and evaluate appropriate responses to their needs. During information gathering, children and adolescents require protection and respect in accordance with the highest ethical standards." This publication draws attention to the many issues which can arise when conducting research with children as participants. The issue of consent and assent is discussed.

http://www.popline.org/docs/1673/299734.html
(accessed 9 May 2008)

Upshur R, Lavery JV, Tindana PO. Taking Tissue Seriously Means Taking Communities Seriously. *BioMedCentral Medical Ethics*, 2007;8:11.

"In this paper, [the authors] outline the salient ethical issues raised by tissue exportation, review the current ethical guidelines and norms, review the literature on what is known empirically about perceptions and practices with respect to tissue exportation from the developing to the developed world, set out what needs to be known in terms of a research agenda, and outline what needs to be done immediately in terms of setting best practices." The authors conclude that any solution will necessitate going beyond concern with individual level consent to meaningful engagement with communities.

http://dx.doi.org/10.1186/1472-6939-8-11
(accessed 25 August 2008)

Wilmshurst P. Scientific Imperialism. *British Medical Journal*, 1997;314:840-841.

"Should research be conducted in a country where the people are unlikely to benefit from the findings because most of the population is too poor to buy effective treatment? Are poor people in developing countries being exploited in research for the benefit of patients in the developed world where subject recruitment to a randomised trial would be difficult?" This editorial addresses questions of inequality arising when health research is conducted in developing countries.

http://www.bmj.com/cgi/content/full/314/7084/840
(accessed 9 May 2008)

IV. Voluntary Informed Consent

Bhutta ZA. Beyond Informed Consent. *Bulletin of the World Health Organization*, 2004, 82:771-777.

"Although a relatively recent phenomenon, the role of informed consent in human research is central to its ethical regulation and conduct. However, guidelines often recommend procedures for obtaining informed consent (usually written consent) that are difficult to implement in developing countries. This paper reviews the guidelines for obtaining informed consent and also discusses prevailing views on current controversies, ambiguities and problems with these guidelines and suggests potential solutions."

http://www.who.int/bulletin/volumes/82/10/771.pdf
(accessed 10 May 2008)

Henderson GE, et al. Clinical Trials and Medical Care: Defining the Therapeutic Misconception. *PLoS Medicine*, 2007; 3(11): 324.

"A key component of informed consent to participate in medical research is the understanding that research is not the same as treatment. However, studies have found that some research participants do not appreciate important differences between research and treatment, a phenomenon called "therapeutic misconception." A consistent definition of therapeutic misconception is missing from the literature, and this hinders attempts to define its prevalence or ways to reduce it. This paper proposes a new definition and describes how it can be operationalized."

http://dx.doi.org/10.1371/journal.pmed.0040324
(accessed 25 August 2008)

Lindegger G, Richter LM. HIV Vaccine Trials: Critical Issues in Informed Consent. *South African Journal of Science*, 2000;96:313-317.

"Informed consent (IC), a fundamental principle of ethics in medical research, is recognized as a vital component of HIV vaccine trials. There are different notions of IC, some legally based and others based on ethics. It is argued that, though legal indemnity is necessary, vaccine trials should be founded on fully ethical considerations." This article explores the differences between the legal and moral arguments for obtaining informed consent from research participants and examines the implications of each before ultimately deciding in favour of a moral or ethical rationale.

http://www.saavi.org.za/lindegger.pdf
(accessed 9 May 2008)

Marshall PA. Ethical Challenges in Study Design and Informed Consent for Health Research in Resource-poor Settings. Geneva, Switzerland: WHO/TDR, 2007.

"This review considers ethical challenges to research design and informed consent in biomedical and behavioural studies conducted in resource-poor settings. A review of the literature explores relevant social, cultural, and ethical issues in the conduct of biomedical and social health research in developing countries. Ten case vignettes illustrate ethical challenges that arise in international research with culturally diverse populations" In addition, this publication offers recommendations to researchers and policy-makers concerned with ethical practices in multinational studies conducted in resource-poor settings. Issues of community consultation, decisional authority to consent, and power inequities are addressed in the context of consent.

https://www.who.int/tdr/publications/tdr-research-publications/ethical-challenges-study-design/pdf/ethical_challenges.pdf
(accessed 30 August 2008)

Molyneux CS, et al. 'Even If They Ask You To Stand By A Tree All Day, You Will Have To Do It (Laughter)…!': Community Voices on the Notion and Practice of Informed Consent for Biomedical Research in Developing Countries. *Social Science and Medicine*, 2005; 61:443-54.

"Ethical dilemmas in biomedical research, especially in vulnerable populations, often spark heated debate. Despite recommendations and guidelines, many issues remain controversial, including the relevance, prioritisation and application of individual voluntary informed consent in non-Western settings. The voices of the people likely to be the subjects of research have been notably absent from the debate." The authors share their findings from discussions with groups of community members living in the rural study area of a large research unit in Kenya. They emphasize that the failure to appreciate the spectrum of views and understandings held by community members risks researchers responding inadequately to the needs and values of those on whom the success of most biomedical research depends.

http://dx.doi.org/10.1016/j.socscimed.2004.12.003
(accessed 25 August 2008)

Préziosi M, et al. Practical Experiences in Obtaining Informed Consent for a Vaccine Trial in Rural Africa. *New England Journal of Medicine*, 1997;336:370-373.

"There is considerable debate about the appropriateness of obtaining individual informed consent in non-Western cultures. In the process of conducting a study of a new pertussis vaccine in a rural community in Senegal, we sought to evaluate the incorporation of clear procedures for obtaining individual informed consent from parents. In this part of Senegal, consent for all previous research with human subjects had been obtained from community leaders on behalf of all eligible members of the community. Individuals could subsequently decline to participate."

http://content.nejm.org/cgi/content/extract/336/5/370
(accessed 25 August 2008)

Rotini C, et al. Community Engagement and Informed Consent in the International Hapmap Project. *Community Genetics*, 2007;10:186-198.

"The International HapMap Consortium has developed the HapMap, a resource that describes the common patterns of human genetic variation (haplotypes). Processes of community/public consultation and individual informed consent were implemented in each locality where samples were collected to understand and attempt to address both individual and group concerns". The experience of approaching genetic variation research in a spirit of openness was a positive one and the authors suggest that this openness can help investigators to "better appreciate the views of the communities whose samples they seek to study and help communities become more engaged in the science."

http://dx.doi.org/10.1159/000101761
(accessed 25 August 2008)

V. Standard of Care

Killen J, et al. Ethics of Clinical Research in the Developing World. *Nature Reviews*, 2002, 2: 210-215.

"Many commentators believe that all clinical trial participants must receive a level of care equivalent to the world's best. Using HIV/AIDS research as an example, [the authors] show how this 'Uniform Care Requirement' can undermine biomedical research aimed at improving global health, and then [they] point towards a more rational and balanced approach to ethical assessment."

http://dx.doi.org/10.1038/nri745
(accessed 25 August 2008)

Kottow MH. Who Is My Brother's Keeper? *Journal of Medical Ethics*, 2002, 28:24-27.

"Recent years have witnessed frequent reports of less stringent ethical standards being applied to both clinical and research medical practices initiated by developed countries in poorer nations. Still more unsettling, a number of articles have endorsed the policy of employing ethical norms in these host countries, which would be unacceptable to both the legislations and the moral standards of the sponsor nations". The author expresses his concern for the support and approval that is being accorded by bioethicists to the application of differential standards.

http://jme.bmj.com/cgi/content/full/28/1/24
(accessed 9 May 2008)

Wolinsky H. The battle of Helsinki: Two Troublesome Paragraphs in the Declaration of Helsinki are Causing a Furor Over Medical Research Ethics. *European Molecular Biology Organization*, 2006 7(7):670-672.

"Later this year, the US Food and Drug Administration plans to rewrite its regulations to eliminate any reference to the Declaration of Helsinki (DoH), a document from the World Medical Association […] that many consider to be the hallmark of medical ethics. This decision, triggered by the 2000 update to the DoH, is the latest move in an increasingly heated debate over medical research ethics. The FDA is reacting in particular to the addition of two controversial paragraphs, which, if adopted in their own regulations, would limit the use of placebos in drug trials and increase the responsibilities of trial sponsors towards research participants." This article presents the arguments and politics concerning the changes to the DoH.

http://dx.doi.org/10.1038/sj.embor.7400743
(accessed 25 August 2008)

VI. Obligations to Participants and to the Community

Andanda PA. Human-Tissue-Related Inventions: Ownership and Intellectual Property Rights in International Collaborative Research in Developing Countries. *Journal of Medical Ethics*, 2008; 34: 3, 171-179.

"There are complex unresolved ethical, legal and social issues related to the use of human tissues obtained in the course of research or diagnostic procedures and retained for further use in research…. It is important for research ethics committees to tread carefully when reviewing research protocols that raise such issues for purposes of ensuring that appropriate benefit sharing agreements, particularly with developing countries, are in place. This paper attempts to analyse the key questions related to ownership and intellectual property rights in commercially viable products derived from human tissue samples."

http://dx.doi.org/10.1136/jme.2006.019612
(accessed 25 August 2008)

Belsky L, Richardson HS. Medical Researchers' Ancillary Clinical Care Responsibilities. *British Medical Journal*, 2004;328:1494-1496.

"Investigation of participants in clinical trials may identify conditions unrelated to the study. Researchers need guidance on whether they have a duty to treat such conditions." Arguing that existing guidelines do not adequately address the ancillary care issues and responsibilities arising during health research, the authors propose an ethical framework that will help delineate researchers' responsibilities.

http://dx.doi.org/10.1136/bmj.328.7454.1494
(accessed 25 August 2008)

MacNeil DS, Fernandez CV. Offering Results to Research Participants. *British Medical Journal*, 2006;332(7535):188.

"Do participants of research trials wish to be offered a summary of the trial results? This practice is being encouraged as a means of demonstrating greater respect for research participants: it recognises the central role of participants in the completion of research studies and avoids treating them as a means to an end." This editorial recognizes the importance of exercising caution and judgment in the provision of individual research results to participants and supports providing results to those who want them.

http://dx.doi.org/10.1136/bmj.332.7535.188
(accessed 25 August 2008)

Participants in the 2001 Conference on Ethical Aspects of Research in Developing Countries. Ethics: fair benefits for research in developing countries. *Science* 2002;298(5601):2133-2134.

"Collaborative, multinational clinical research, especially between developed and developing countries, has been the subject of controversy. Much of this attention has focused on the standard of care used in randomized trials. Much less discussed, but probably more important in terms of its impact on health, is the claim that, in order to avoid exploitation, interventions proven safe and effective through research in developing countries should be made "reasonably available" in those countries."

http://dx.doi.org/10.1126/science.1076899
(accessed 9 May 2008)

Potts M. Thinking About Vaginal Microbicide Testing. *American Journal of Public Health*. 2000;90(2).

"A vaginal microbicide could slow the spread of HIV. To date, volunteers in placebo-controlled trials of candidate microbicides have been counseled to use condoms. This does not reduce the number of volunteers exposed to possible risk, but shifts the allotment of risk from those conducting the trial to those women who may be least able to make autonomous decisions. Alternative ways of meeting the obligation to offer volunteers active benefits are explored." This controversial article challenges accepted practice and generated numerous responses on the issue of condom provision and counseling in microbicide trials.

http://www.pubmedcentral.nih.gov/articlerender.fcgi?artid=1446143 (accessed 17 April 2008)

Shapiro K, Benatar SR. HIV Prevention Research and Global Inequality: Steps Towards Improved Standards of Care. *Journal of Medical Ethics Online* 2005;31:39-47.

"Intensification of poverty and degradation of health infrastructure over recent decades in countries most affected by HIV/AIDS present formidable challenges to clinical research. This paper addresses the overall standard of health care (SOC) that should be provided to research participants in developing countries, rather than the narrow definition of SOC that has characterized the international debate on standards of health care. It argues that contributing to sustainable improvements in health by progressively ratcheting the standard of care upwards for research participants and their communities is an ethical obligation of those in resource-rich countries who sponsor and implement research in poorer ones."

http://jme.bmj.com/cgi/reprint/31/1/39
(accessed 17 April 2008)

Simon C, Mosavel M, van Stade D. Ethical Challenges in the Design and Conduct of Locally Relevant International Health Research. *Social Science and Medicine*, 2007;64(9):1960-1969.

"In this paper, [the authors] consider some of the challenges associated with the ethical need to conduct locally relevant international health research. We examine a cervical cancer research initiative in a resource-poor community in South Africa, and consider the extent to which this research was relevant to the expressed needs and concerns of community members."

http://dx.doi.org/10.1016/j.socscimed.2007.01.009
(accessed 25 August 2008)

Tarantola D, et al. Ethical Considerations Related to the Provision of Care and Treatment in Vaccine Trials. *Vaccine*, 2007, 25:4863-4874.

"Ethical principles of beneficence and justice combined with international human rights norms and standards create certain obligations on researchers, sponsors and public health authorities.[…] However, these obligations are poorly defined in practical terms, inconsistently understood or inadequately applied. The present document addresses specifically the setting of standards applicable to care and treatment in vaccine trials […] and proposes a structured approach to consensual decision making in the context of the clinical trial of vaccines." The paper is based on a series of global consultations initiated by WHO and UNAIDS.

http://dx.doi.org/10.1016/j.vaccine.2007.03.022
(accessed 25 August 2008)

Zong Z. Should Post-trial Provision of Beneficial Experimental Interventions be Mandatory in Developing Countries? *Journal of Medical Ethics*, 2008;34:188-192.

"The need for continuing provision of beneficial experimental interventions after research is concluded remains a controversial topic in bioethics for research….This paper summarises recommendations from international and national guidelines. Ethical principles and practical issues relating to post-trial provision are also discussed. In conclusion, post-trial provision is not necessary in all situations and a set of criteria are proposed to identify the situations that beneficial interventions should be provided beyond the research period. However, mandatory post-trial supply of beneficial experimental interventions should be assured for those who still need and are able to benefit from them but have no alternative access."

http://dx.doi.org/10.1136/jme.2006.018754
(accessed 25 August 2008)

VII. Privacy and Confidentiality

Shalowitz DI, Miller FG. Disclosing Individual Results of Clinical Research. *Journal of the American Medical Association*, 2005; 294:6:737-740.

This paper discusses the responsibility of investigators to communicate the results of research to study participants. The author argues that "disclosure of individual results should be addressed in all research involving human participants."

http://jama.ama-assn.org/cgi/content/full/294/6/737
(accessed 9 May 2008)

Lawlor DA, Stone T. Public Health and Data Protection: An Inevitable Collision or Potential for a Meeting of Minds? *International Journal of Epidemiology*, 2001; 30:1221-1225.

This paper reviews current data protection legislation and guidance, looking at its consequences on public health practices. In addition, it discusses recent changes to legislation and guidance in relation to established medical principles.

http://ije.oxfordjournals.org/cgi/content/full/30/6/1221
(accessed 9 May 2008)

VIII. Professional Ethics

Bodenheimer T. Conflict of Interest in Clinical Drug Trials: a Risk Factor for Scientific Misconduct. (2000)

"In clinical drug trials, conflict of interest usually refers to the situation in which an investigator has a financial relationship (often research funding) with a company whose product the investigator is studying. There is nothing intrinsically wrong with conflicts of interest; they are virtually ubiquitous in clinical drug trials because so many trials are funded by the manufacturer of the product being studied. The problem is less conflict of interest itself; the problem is that conflict of interest may be a risk factor for scientific misconduct."

http://www.hhs.gov/ohrp/coi/bodenheimer.htm
(accessed 9 May 2008)

Campbell EG, et al. Financial Relationships Between Institutional Review Board Member and Industry. *New England Journal of Medicine*, 2006; 355(22): 2321-2329.

"Little is known about the nature, extent, and consequences of financial relationships between industry and institutional review board (IRB) members in academic institutions. [The authors] surveyed IRB members about such relationships and [conclude that] relationships between IRB members and industry are common, and members sometimes participate in decisions about protocols sponsored by companies with which they have a financial relationship. Current regulations and policies should be examined to be sure that there is an appropriate way to handle conflicts of interest stemming from relationships with industry."

http://content.nejm.org/cgi/content/full/355/22/2321
(accessed 10 May 2008)

Faunce TA, Jeffrys S. Whistleblowing and Scientific Misconduct: Renewing Legal and Virtue Ethics Foundations. *Medicine and Law*, 2007;26(3):567-584.

"Whistleblowing in relation to scientific research misconduct, despite the benefits of increased transparency and accountability it often has brought to society and the discipline of science itself, remains generally regarded as a pariah activity by many of the most influential relevant organizations. The motivations of whistleblowers and those supporting them continued to be questioned and their actions criticised by colleagues and management, despite statutory protections for reasonable disclosures appropriately made in good faith and for the public interest."

http://www.ncbi.nlm.nih.gov/pubmed/17970253
abstract only (accessed 10 May 2008)

Momen H, Gollogly L. Cross-cultural Perspectives of Scientific Misconduct. *Medicine and Law*, 2007;26(3): 409-416.

"The increasing globalization of scientific research lends urgency to the need for international agreement on the concepts of scientific misconduct. Universal spiritual and moral principles on which ethical standards are generally based indicate that it is possible to reach international agreement on the ethical principles underlying good scientific practice [...] Defining scientific misconduct to be universally recognized and universally sanctioned means addressing the broader question of ensuring that research is not only well-designed – and addresses a real need for better evidence – but that it is ethically conducted in different cultures".

http://www.ncbi.nlm.nih.gov/pubmed/17970242
abstract only (accessed 10 May 2008).

Appendix

The ethical principles included here are reprinted from the *International Ethical Guidelines for Biomedical Research Involving Human Subjects*, prepared by the Council for International Organizations of Medical Sciences (CIOMS) in collaboration with the World Health Organization.[1] While these principles are widely known and referred to, it is important to recognize that there are additional and alternative principles that provide useful conceptual and practical frameworks.

GENERAL ETHICAL PRINCIPLES

All research involving human subjects should be conducted in accordance with three basic ethical principles, namely respect for persons, beneficence and justice. It is generally agreed that these principles, which in the abstract have equal moral force, guide the conscientious preparation of proposals for scientific studies. In varying circumstances they may be expressed differently and given different moral weight, and their application may lead to different decisions or courses of action. The [CIOMS] guidelines are directed at the application of these principles to research involving human subjects.

Respect for persons incorporates at least two fundamental ethical considerations, namely:

a respect for autonomy, which requires that those who are capable of deliberation about their personal choices should be treated with respect for their capacity for self-determination; and

b protection of persons with impaired or diminished autonomy, which requires that those who are dependent or vulnerable be afforded security against harm or abuse.

Beneficence refers to the ethical obligation to maximize benefits and to minimize harms. This principle gives rise to norms requiring that the risks of research be reasonable in the light of the expected benefits, that the research design be sound, and that the investigators be competent both to conduct the research and to safeguard the welfare of the research subjects. Beneficence further proscribes the deliberate infliction of harm on persons; this aspect of beneficence is sometimes expressed as a separate principle, **nonmaleficence** (do no harm).

Justice refers to the ethical obligation to treat each person in accordance with what is morally right and proper, to give each person what is due to him or her. In the ethics of research involving human subjects the principle refers primarily to distributive justice, which requires the equitable distribution of both the burdens and the benefits of participation in research. Differences in distribution of burdens and benefits are justifiable only if they are based on morally relevant distinctions between persons; one such distinction is vulnerability. "Vulnerability" refers to a substantial incapacity to protect one's own interests owing to such impediments as lack of capability to give informed consent, lack of alternative means of obtaining medical care or other expensive necessities, or being a junior or subordinate member of a hierarchical group. Accordingly, special provision must be made for the protection of the rights and welfare of vulnerable persons.

Sponsors of research or investigators cannot, in general, be held accountable for unjust conditions where the research is conducted, but they must refrain from practices that are likely to worsen unjust conditions or contribute to new inequities. Neither should they take advantage of the relative inability of low-resource countries or vulnerable populations to protect their own interests, by conducting research inexpensively and avoiding complex regulatory systems of industrialized countries in order to develop products for the lucrative markets of those countries.

---

[1] These ethical principles are reprinted in full and with permission from the *International Ethical Guidelines for Biomedical Research Involving Human Subjects*, prepared by the Council for International Organizations of Medical Sciences (CIOMS) in collaboration with the World Health Organization, Geneva: 2002. http://www.cioms.ch (accessed 9 May 2008)

In general, the research project should leave low-resource countries or communities better off than previously or, at least, no worse off. It should be responsive to their health needs and priorities in that any product developed is made reasonably available to them, and as far as possible leave the population in a better position to obtain effective health care and protect its own health.

Justice requires also that the research be responsive to the health conditions or needs of vulnerable subjects. The subjects selected should be the least vulnerable necessary to accomplish the purposes of the research. Risk to vulnerable subjects is most easily justified when it arises from interventions or procedures that hold out for them the prospect of direct health-related benefit. Risk that does not hold out such prospect must be justified by the anticipated benefit to the population of which the individual research subject is representative.

300028